STAND-UP
PADDLE-
BOARDING
IN GREAT BRITAIN

STAND-UP PADDLE- BOARDING IN GREAT BRITAIN

BEAUTIFUL PLACES TO PADDLEBOARD
IN ENGLAND, SCOTLAND & WALES

JO MOSELEY

Vertebrate Publishing, Sheffield
www.adventurebooks.com

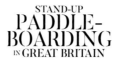

STAND-UP PADDLE-BOARDING IN GREAT BRITAIN

BEAUTIFUL PLACES TO PADDLEBOARD IN ENGLAND, SCOTLAND & WALES

First published in 2022 by Vertebrate Publishing.

VERTEBRATE PUBLISHING
Omega Court, 352 Cemetery Road, Sheffield S11 8FT, United Kingdom.
www.adventurebooks.com

A CIP catalogue record for this book is available from the British Library.

ISBN 978-1-83981-149-4 (Paperback)
ISBN 978-1-83981-150-0 (Ebook)

Front cover: Cal Major paddleboarding at Lower Lode,
near Tewkesbury on the River Severn © @jamesappletonphotography
Back cover: L–R: Sunrise at Runswick Bay © Charlotte Graham; A peaceful paddle on the River Dee; A sunny day
on London's Regent's Canal; Ullswater in the Lake District; The red cliffs at Sidmouth; The beautiful Afon Teifi;
A #2MinuteBeachClean; Looking over Aberporth.

Photography by Jo Moseley except where otherwise credited.

Mapping contains OS data © Crown copyright and database right (2022)
and Openstreetmap.org data © OpenStreetMap contributors.
Cartography by Richard Ross, Active Maps Ltd. www.activemaps.co.uk

Edited by Jess McElhattan, cover design by Jane Beagley, layout and production by Rosie Edwards.
www.adventurebooks.com

Printed and bound in Europe by Latitude Press.

Vertebrate Publishing is committed to printing on paper from sustainable sources.

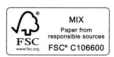

Every effort has been made to achieve accuracy of the information in this guidebook. The author, publishers and
copyright owners can take no responsibility for: loss or injury (including fatal) to persons; loss or damage to property
or equipment; trespass, irresponsible behaviour or any other mishap that may be suffered as a result of following the
route descriptions or advice offered in this guidebook. The inclusion of a track or path as part of a route, or otherwise
recommended, in this guidebook does not guarantee that the track or path will remain a right of way. If conflict with
landowners arises we advise that you act politely and leave by the shortest route available. If the matter needs to be
taken further then please take it up with the relevant authority.

SAFETY STATEMENT

Stand-up paddleboarding and wild swimming are activities that carry a risk of personal injury or death. Participants must
be aware of and accept that these risks are present and they should be responsible for their own actions and involvement.
Nobody involved in the writing and production of this guidebook accepts any responsibility for any errors that it may
contain, or are they liable for any injuries or damage that may arise from its use. Stand-up paddleboarding, outdoor
swimming and particularly wild swimming are inherently dangerous and the fact that individual descriptions in this volume
do not point out such dangers does not mean that they do not exist. Take care.

Opposite The Aldford Iron Bridge on the River Dee, Llyn Tegid © Caroline Dawson (SUP Lass Paddle Adventures)

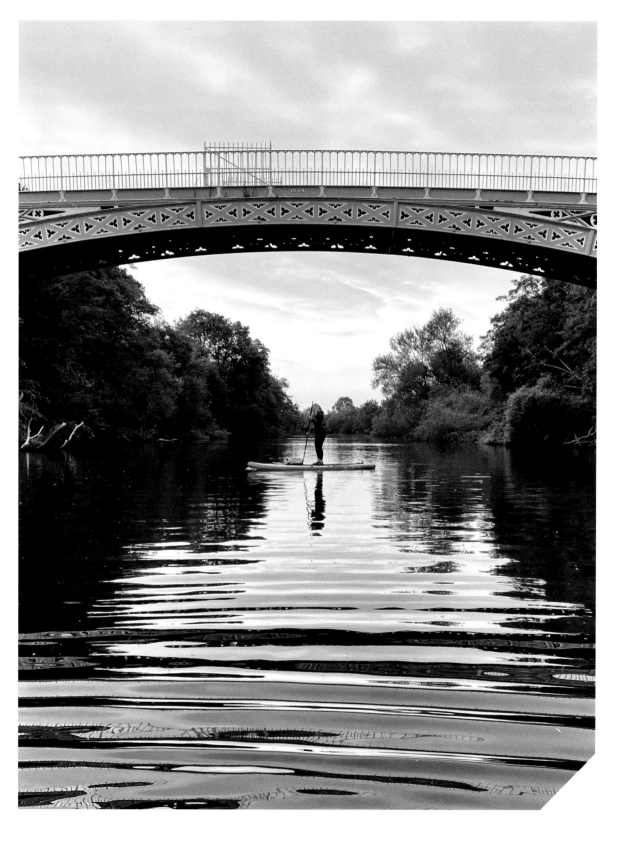

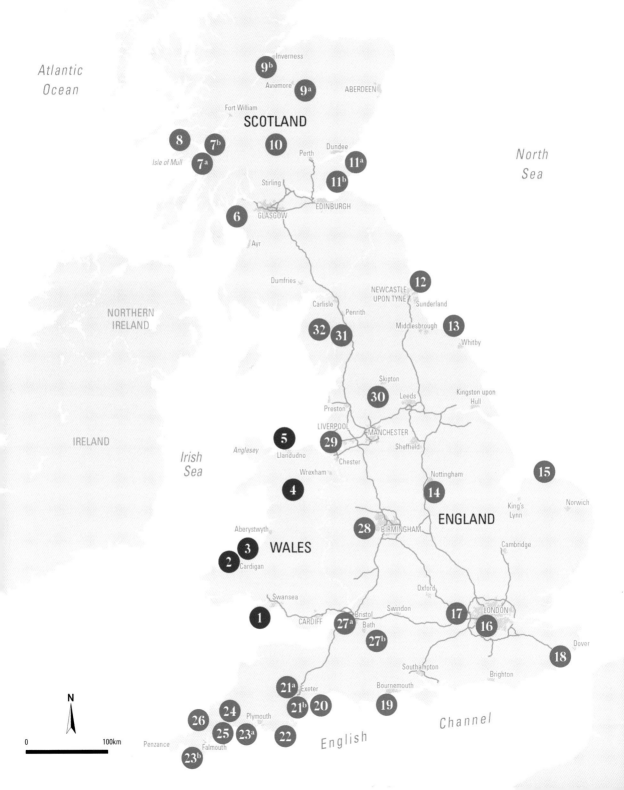

Introduction ix

**The history and growth of SUP x How to get started in SUP xi
Equipment and kit xvi Safety xix Planning xix Weather xxi
Being environmentally thoughtful and responsible xxiii
How I decided which places to include xxv**

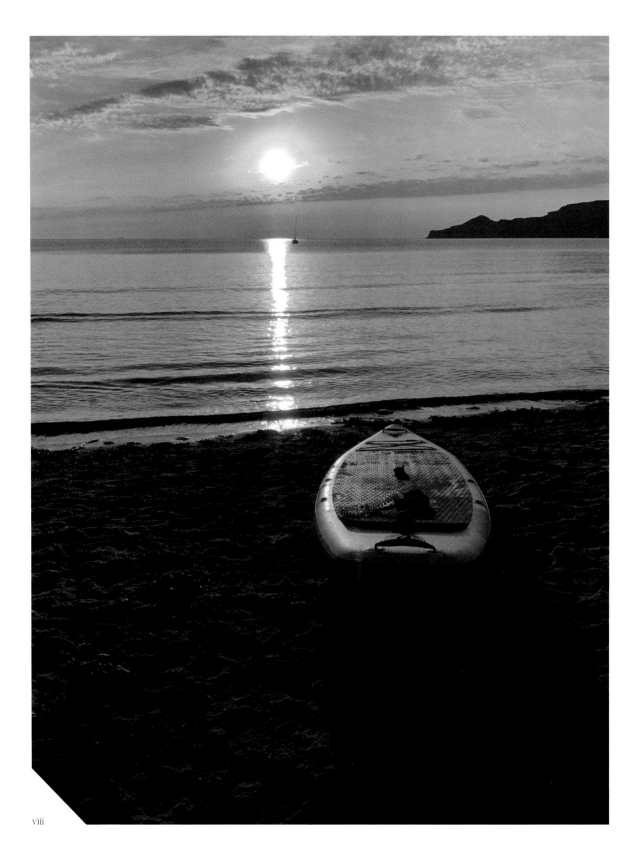

Opposite Sunrise at Runswick Bay

Introduction

'Do you remember how it felt the first time you went paddleboarding?'

This is a question I ask all my guests on my podcast, *The Joy of SUP – The Paddleboarding Sunshine Podcast*. For almost all, that moment is fresh in their memory.

In a world that makes so many demands upon us each day, with little time to simply be, stand-up paddleboarding (SUP) has given so many of us the opportunity to be a beginner once more, to fall and try again and to celebrate the small steps along the way. We have found friendships and freedom, learned that maybe we are stronger and more courageous than we thought and that there is adventure on our doorstep if we pause to look around. A chance to walk on water and, I hope, appreciate that we all belong there too.

I shall never forget my first time on a paddleboard on 24 September 2016 in the Lake District. From the moment I stood up and looked out across Derwent Water, I knew that this was something special. I had injured my knee at the beginning of the year, and my spirits and sense of joy were dulled by months of pain. In September, I set myself a challenge to spend 30 minutes each day moving outside. 'For the first time in months, I felt like a warrior, not a worrier,' is how I describe that afternoon. Yes, I fell and yes, I doubted myself as we made our way across the water, but I also smiled and laughed more than I had in months. Two months later I chose my first paddleboard for my fifty-second birthday present, a white, blue and orange Starboard Astro Zen that I still sometimes ride today. And so began my love story with paddleboarding.

In the years since, SUP has helped me navigate life with greater hope through grief, loss, anxiety, a difficult menopause, flying solo with my sons and being an empty nester. I have written articles, made tiny award-winning films (*Found at Sea* and *Finding Joy)* and launched my podcast celebrating the paddleboarding community.

In 2019 I became the first woman, aged 54, to SUP coast to coast across Northern England, picking up litter and raising money for the surf therapy charity The Wave Project and 2 Minute Foundation. A film about my journey, created with Frit Tam of Passion Fruit Pictures, *Brave Enough – A Journey Home to Joy*, has been screened at prestigious film festivals and online to a warm reception and critical acclaim.

Paddleboarding has brought a sense of community, joy, strength and purpose that I had forgotten was possible outside my roles as a mother, daughter, sister and friend. My connection to the environment has deepened, as has my commitment to look after the waterways that bring such happiness. I never claim to be the fastest, strongest or fittest paddleboarder; I have watched in awe the technical skills of those who have so generously shared their time with me as I researched this book.

My goal with *Stand-up Paddleboarding in Great Britain* is to share these possibilities of place and people with you. You'll meet paddleboarding friends and heroes and explore the magic of the rivers, lakes, lochs, harbours, beaches, canals and coasts that they are lucky enough to call home. Without exception, every place I visited and bring to you here surpassed my expectations and I returned richer for the experience.

I hope *Stand-up Paddleboarding in Great Britain* will spark your curiosity to discover new destinations in England, Scotland and Wales and also to find adventure on your doorstep on waterways that perhaps, like me, you have overlooked in the past. Whether you are a beginner or a more seasoned SUP enthusiast, my wish is that there is somewhere here for you, and that you will feel the same sense of wonder I feel putting on my leash and setting forth on my board.

On her podcast *How to Fail With Elizabeth Day*, author and presenter Elizabeth Day shared the advice of acclaimed novelist Maggie O'Farrell: 'the best writing you can do is the writing you can't not do,' she said, 'you have to tell the story that is bursting to be told.'

Writing this book has been one of the greatest honours of my life. I truly hope I have done justice to the stories of place and people that I feel are bursting to be told.

For more information on the topics covered in the following pages, go to *www.adventurebooks.com/blogs/blog/stand-up-paddleboarding-information*

Key

📍 Entry point

📍 Exit point

📍 Combined exit and entry point

🔄 Turn around point (the point of the route at which you start heading back to your launch location)

🚌 Public transport – bus

🚆 Public transport – rail

Ⓔ Underground

Ⓜ Metro

Ⓟ Parking

The history and growth of SUP

Over the last few years, paddleboarding and the SUP community have grown hugely. According to British Canoeing, the number of its members who tick SUP as their main interest has grown by 229 per cent from October 2019. It is the fastest-growing discipline within its membership. Of the SUP paddlers, 51 per cent are female, and 73 per cent of its SUP membership is between 30 and 60 years old.

I have always wondered when SUP as a sport came to Britain, and so with the help of SUP writer Sarah Thornely I contacted two early enthusiasts, Simon Bassett and Brian Johncey. Simon is chairman and joint head coach of British Stand Up Paddleboarding Association (BSUPA) and owner of SUP school 2XS, who began SUP in 2006. At that time he believes there were fewer than 10 people paddling in the UK. A year later he set up BSUPA, training instructors and setting up the BSUPA national

SUP race series. Brian Johncey, owner of Blue Chip Board Store, also started SUP around this time. The Blue Chip paddlers were the first on the River Thames at Hampton Court in 2007. In 2011 he organised a SUP racing event, the Battle of the Thames, with 48 competitors. By 2019 the numbers had risen to over 200. He says recreational SUP really took off in 2014, and that this accounts for 95 per cent of his board sales.

I feel honoured to hear these experiences, and if you know any others who can shed light on the history of SUP in the UK please do let me know. In the meantime, Steve West's book *Stand Up Paddle: A paddlers' guide* offers research and insight into the history of the sport worldwide.

It's also interesting to reflect that if you are taking up SUP today, you really are still at the start of things; we are all part of this exciting journey together.

How to get started in SUP

One of the attractions of paddleboarding, especially for anyone new to water sports, is its simplicity and accessibility. However, whenever we are near or on a body of water there are risks and challenges to think about. This is not just for our own safety and enjoyment, but the safety of other water users around us and the emergency services that would need to rescue us if something goes wrong.

In this section, I will go through a few ideas to think about when you get started with SUP and give you links to more specialised information to build up your knowledge and skills, and ultimately make SUP even more fun.

The basics

For those new to SUP, there can be a lot to take in. Here is a list of some of the equipment you will encounter:

» **Inflatable board** – inflatable boards are ones that you pump up yourself, by hand or using an electric pump. When not in use, they are deflated, rolled up and packed away for transport and storage. They usually come as a package with a bag, paddle and a pump to inflate them. Also known as iSUPs.

» **Hardboard** – also known as rigid or solid boards, hardboards are usually made of fibre glass and epoxy resin wrapped around a foam core. They can be made in shapes and sizes more suited to specialist SUP disciplines such as racing or surfing. They do not fold down and you do not need to inflate them.

» **Paddle** – this is like a handheld oar that you use to move through the water. It has a handle, shaft and blade: the blade is the part that goes into the water.

» **Leash** – this attaches you to your board and can be worn around your ankle, calf or around the waist. Your board is a good buoyancy aid and wearing a leash means you won't be separated from it should you

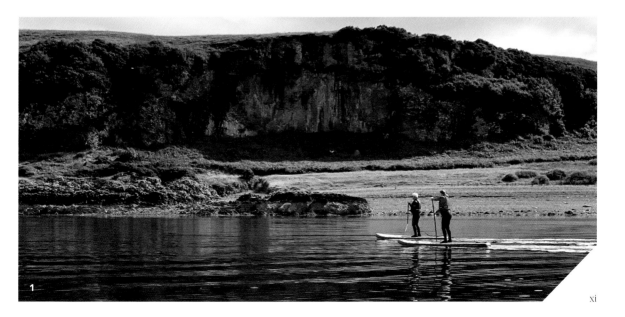

fall in. For recreational paddles, such as the ones shared in this guide, a coiled leash is recommended. SUP surfers would wear a straight leash. It is important to keep up to date with leash advice.

» **Buoyancy aid** – a piece of equipment that will keep a conscious person who is able to keep their head above water afloat. Also known as personal flotation devices (PFDs).

» **Fin** – fins are attached to the back (tail) of your board to help with control, direction and balance. The number and size of the fins (for example, a centre fin and two side fins) on a board can vary according to the make and type of board as well as what sort of paddling you will be doing.

Choosing an instructor

My number one top tip for anyone getting into SUP is to take a lesson or course of lessons with a qualified instructor.

They cover safety, skills, equipment, the environment and confidence building; everything from what to wear and how to set up your board to SUP strokes, turns and stopping, what to do if you fall off and how to self-rescue.

Additionally, they might share knowledge of the local SUP spots. A SUP school, club or instructor may also run SUP socials where you'll meet other people from the paddleboarding community. It's worth investing in some lessons if you've been paddling for a while but didn't have chance to have a lesson at the outset. A good instructor will be more than happy to review your technique and help you build up your skills and knowledge.

In addition to taking lessons with a qualified instructor, you could also consider online safety skills courses, for example the Water Skills Academy's (WSA) safety video tutorials and iSUP Smart online course, the *SUPfm* SUP Safety Course and British Canoeing's Go Paddling website for SUP safety video tutorials. I have also listed some instructional books in the further reading pages (p211).

Learning and improving your skills, knowledge and understanding of the environments you'll paddle in will help make you safer and more confident of your ability to judge conditions every time you are on the water. This in turn will make it much more fun.

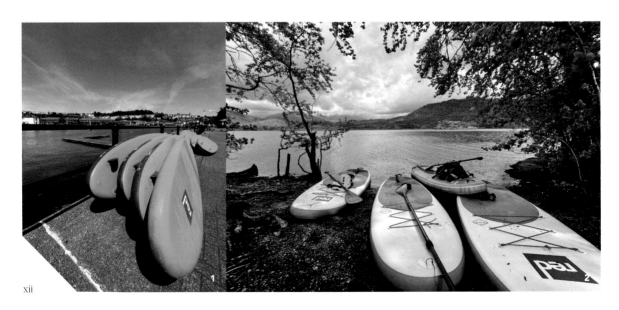

1 Paddleboards in the sunshine at Bristol Harbour   **2** Looking out to Derwent Water

CHOOSING A QUALIFIED INSTRUCTOR

Most instructors and schools will put their qualifications and accreditations on their website or social media details. If you don't see that information, feel free to ask. Awarding bodies they may have trained with are the Academy of Surfing Instructors (ASI), British Canoeing (or a British Canoeing affiliated club), BSUPA, International Surfing Association (ISA) or WSA.

Licensing and access
PADDLING ON INLAND WATERWAYS

If you're wondering whether you can paddle anywhere you want on inland waterways, the short answer is no. There are over 68,000 kilometres of inland waterways in England and Wales. Of that, approximately 2,250 kilometres can be paddled uncontested, which equates to four per cent. This is why British Canoeing is developing the *Clear Access, Clear Waters* campaign working for 'fair, shared and sustainable open access on water for all'. As Ben Seal of British Canoeing explained to me, only a small percentage of waterways in England (and even fewer in Wales) have a Statutory Right of Navigation. British Canoeing has been campaigning for a change in the law and supporting paddlers to be proactive in paddling responsibly, respecting the environment and other users and demonstrating that they are guardians of our waters.

LICENCES

In England and Wales, you need a licence to paddleboard on inland waterways (such as river navigations and canals) managed by the Canal & River Trust and Environment Agency, plus others such as the Norfolk Broads. You can buy a licence from British Canoeing, Canoe Wales, the Canal & River Trust, the WSA or directly from some navigation authorities. When deciding where to buy your licence, look at what and where is covered plus the benefits, for

example liability insurance included within the membership fee, and which is right for you.

In Scotland, you do not need a licence to paddleboard due to the Land Reform (Scotland) Act 2003. However, membership of the Scottish Canoe Association offers a number of benefits including liability insurance.

ADDITIONAL CHARGES

Some places such as the Royal Military Canal (p119) and Liverpool's Royal Albert Dock (p185) require an extra fee as well as a licence. Harbours may require a licence from the Harbour Master's Office. Some lakes are private and charge a launch fee so do check ahead.

Before you travel somewhere new, do your research so you have the right information and can explore with confidence. Visit *www.gopaddling.info* to see which, if any, licence is required.

Choosing your equipment
DECIDING ON YOUR BOARD

Buying your own paddleboard is a big decision, both financially and as an investment in your well-being; you want to get it right. I asked Sean and Claire Scott from The New Forest Paddle Sport Company for their advice:

» **Construction** – consider whether you want a hard or inflatable paddleboard. Hardboards give a better paddling experience due to a shaped and more refined board, but are heavier than most inflatables and are difficult to transport and store. Inflatable boards are lightweight and robust and normally come as a package with pumps, paddles and bags, but are limited in performance paddling or trickier conditions due to board shaping.

» **Location** – consider what type of paddling you want to do and where. There are lots of different boards designed for a range of activities, from SUP surfing, touring and racing to SUP yoga.

» **Particular boards** – consider what you want your board to do. If you are new to SUP and want a board that will do everything, an all-round-style board may suit you best. Be aware, however, that these are slower and not manoeuvrable enough for large waves. If you want to go on river paddling tours or day trips, a touring-designed board is longer and narrower for increased glide and efficiency over distance. If you want to tour on a river or canal with lots of portaging (carrying) or do one-way trips then inflatables are easier to carry and pack away. For coastal paddling on day trips, hard touring boards will handle the chop and swell better than an inflatable.

Tips for inflatable boards

» In hot weather, let some of the air out of your inflatable board and keep the board out of direct heat and sunlight. Simply pump it up when you are about to go on the water.

» Whether you use an electric pump or handpump is a preference and I personally enjoy the ritual of pumping up my board.

» Do not be surprised that when you deflate an inflatable board it can be very loud. As a courtesy to people around me in a public place I try and warn them that I am about to deflate.

» Investing in an upgraded paddle will have a positive impact on your technique, endurance and comfort.

CHOOSING A PADDLE

It is important when buying packages to look at all the accessories and their quality, especially with paddles. The best thing you can do is try out lots of different paddles and boards before purchasing your first board:

» **Material** – the more expensive packages come with carbon paddles and high-quality pumps and bags which will last. The cheaper packages tend to come with aluminium paddles which can corrode quickly in saltwater, don't always float and are heavy.

» **Shape** – the shape of a paddle is very important as well as the size: standard blade shapes are the classic teardrop or the High Aspect shape, which is designed for racing and touring and will give you a more efficient paddle stroke.

I spoke with Claire Scott recently and learned that approximately 90 to 95 per cent of new boards purchased at her shop are inflatable. I use an inflatable board as I simply don't have the space at home to store a hardboard. Almost everyone I paddled with researching the book used an inflatable too.

COILED LEASHES

A leash is a vital part of your safety equipment. If you fall in the water, the leash means your board will remain nearby. Leashes can be straight (used in SUP surf) or coiled. Most recreational SUP packages are currently supplied with a coiled leash, which is worn around your calf or ankle. The leash sits on the deck (or top) of the board so that there is less chance it will snag on branches, ropes, moorings or obstructions under the surface. A coiled leash can also be used with a quick-release (or QR) belt, which is worn around your waist. The QR belt has a buckle and a pull cord or toggle. It sits high out of the water and is less likely to snag on debris on moving water, as you find on estuaries or rivers.

You may find yourself in a situation where you need to separate yourself from your board, where there is a risk of entrapment on an obstruction. A QR belt will allow you to free yourself by pulling the toggle at your waist rather than trying to reach down to your ankle, which could be difficult if the force of the water is pushing you down.

Some brands sell QR belts with their boards, but they are available to buy separately. At the time of writing, a campaign is calling for manufacturers to supply them as standard. My preference is to now wear a QR belt.

Tips for leashes

» There is very specific advice for SUP surfing and white water SUP. It is important you follow the guidelines for these disciplines.
» Have a lesson with a qualified instructor or coach, learn how to use a QR correctly and practise on land.
» Ensure that you fix your leash correctly and securely to your paddleboard each time you use it.
» Regularly check your leash for decay and potential breakage.
» Keep up to date with safety and equipment advice from platforms such as ASI, British Canoeing, BSUPA, ISA, WSA, Stand Up Paddle UK, the RNLI, RLSS and *SUP Mag UK*.

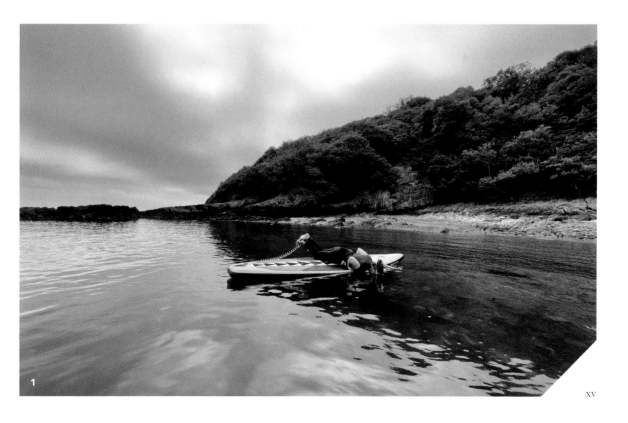

Equipment and kit

When you start SUP it can be daunting looking at the different options available, and what works for someone else might not work for you. The questions I ask myself before buying or choosing what to wear are:

» Where am I paddling?
» What type of paddling am I doing?
» What are the air and water temperatures and wider weather conditions?
» How likely am I to fall in, based on my experience, skills and the body of water?
» Is it comfortable, do I like it and will it allow me to paddle freely?
» What is my budget and how often will I use this piece of kit?
» What is it made of and how sustainable is it?

Remember that this book does not include SUP surfing, where a wetsuit is best, or white water SUP, where you will need specialist equipment.

I spoke with Ben Longhurst at WSA who recommends focusing on preparing for the water temperature, not the air temperature, each season. For example, in winter both air and water temperatures will be cold, but in spring the air temperature will be warming up but the water temperature will still be cold if you fall in.

» **Basic kit** – your basic outerwear for paddleboarding should be swimwear, quick-dry leggings, a rash vest, neoprene leggings and a top or a thin wetsuit. Even in summer you may need a windproof or neoprene jacket. Remember a cap or hat to protect you from the sun and long sleeves on your wetsuit or rash vest. In the autumn or spring you might add a cagoule, warm sweaters, waterproof trousers or a thicker wetsuit. In winter you may also add a warm hat and gloves.

» **Footwear** – think about where your launch point is, how you will launch and exit, what obstacles there might be and what you might step on if you fall in, particularly on canals or rivers. Different options would be wetsuit socks or boots with a hard sole, aqua shoes, trainers or waterproof shoes. It's lovely to paddle barefoot on your board on the sea, however, think about where you will launch and exit as well as returning to your car.

» **Gloves** – don't forget to keep your hands warm with neoprene, woolly or waterproof gloves. You can buy neoprene mitts which have a hole in, so you are still connected to your board.

» **Wetsuits and neoprene options** – a typical wetsuit has long arms and legs, but you may prefer a shortie (a wetsuit with short arms and legs) or a Long John or Jane (a full wetsuit with no arms). A thinner, summer wetsuit might be referred to as 3/2 or 4/3, which means the body of the wetsuit is three millimetres or four millimetres thick and the arms and legs two millimetres or three millimetres. This gives you the warmth where you need it around your torso and the flexibility on your arms and legs for movement. A thicker, winter wetsuit might be referred to as a 5/4, which means the body of the wetsuit is five millimetres and the arms and legs four millimetres.

» **Dry trousers and dry suits** – if you plan to paddle regularly throughout the colder months, you could look at investing in dry trousers and a jacket or an all-in-one dry suit. These may also have built-in socks, over which you then wear boots. Remember if you choose this option to get bigger boots to accommodate the sock and any layers you wear underneath.

» **Changing robes and mats** – a changing robe will allow you to change and keep you cosy after you have been on the water. A changing mat is helpful to change on a rough surface, especially important if you have dry suit trousers with socks which you don't want to rip.
» **Extras** – many paddlers put leashes, extra fins, gloves, boots and any wet gear in a large plastic laundry basket so it is all in one place.

Tips for essential outerwear
» **It is better to take an extra layer and not need it than be chilly without one.**
» **Think how far you will be from a change of clothes if you fall in.**
» **A vest-style buoyancy aid adds an extra layer of warmth.**

BUOYANCY AIDS

Another key part of your safety equipment is your PFD or buoyancy aid. There are two styles: chest/vest or waist belt. I prefer a vest style with a zip.

» **Chest/vest** – a vest style that has a snug fit and allows you to move your arms. Check that it is not too bulky at the front, which might make getting back on the board tricky if you fall in. Some brands also make PFDs that are a better fit for women.
» **Waist belt** – contains an inflatable bladder and small gas cylinder, released by pulling the toggle. You can also manually top it up with a valve. You will need to replace the gas cylinder if you use it in an emergency. There is a waterproof storage pocket at the front. Palm make one called the Glide and Red and the Airbelt PFD.

CLEANING YOUR KIT

Cleaning your board, paddle and leashes regularly not only keeps them in good condition so that they last longer, but is also important from an environmental viewpoint. Rinsing with fresh, cold water and then allowing them to dry completely after each session is good practice. I also clean my board with an eco-friendly scrub, such as SUP Scrub. Hardboards will need more specialised maintenance and repair.

What to take on your paddleboard

I spoke with Ben at WSA for his thoughts on what to carry on our boards. The exact items you need to take will depend on the type of journey, when and where you are going and the weather forecast.

» **Fully charged phone in a waterproof case** – keep the phone close to you, perhaps round your neck on a lanyard, rather than in your dry bag where you might not be able to reach it in an emergency. Always tell someone before you go out where you are going and what time you intend to return, especially if you are paddling alone.
» **Dry bag** – attached safely to your board or one you wear like a rucksack. I have a smaller dry bag containing keys and a battery pack for my phone.
» **A drink** – you will be surprised how dehydrated you can become paddleboarding and your judgement and ability will be impaired.
» **'Pea-less' whistle** – to attract attention.
» **Throw bag and line.**
» **Snacks** – I prefer to use a reusable plastic or tin box or beeswax wraps, rather than single-use plastic bags.
» **Hand sanitiser** – to use before eating.
» **Extra clothing** – a hat, cap, gloves, an extra layer of warmth, cagoule in case of rain and a change of clothes.

1 The fins of a paddleboard
2 A sea urchin on Ganavan Sands

» Sunscreen and sunglasses – with floating straps.
» Torch.
» Knife.
» Spare fin and fin bolt – if this is how your fin is fitted to your board. Also a spare leash, paddle and pump.
» First aid kit – just to cover blisters, cuts, stings and other minor scrapes.
» Repair kit – some duct tape, cable ties and cord can repair most things, from leashes to paddles, to keep you moving.
» Litter picker and bag – to do a #2MinuteBeachClean.
» Mask and snorkel.
» Personal locator beacon or flare – for an emergency on longer adventure touring and coastal trips. You may also want to take a VHF radio qualification.
» Space blanket or emergency shelter – for longer adventures.

Tips for what to take

» Write your name and phone details on your board on a sticker or in permanent marker. If you're separated from your board while paddling on the coast, this will allow the coastguard to contact you and avoid an air-and-sea search operation being launched. You may also get your board back.
» Keep spare clothes and food in the car.

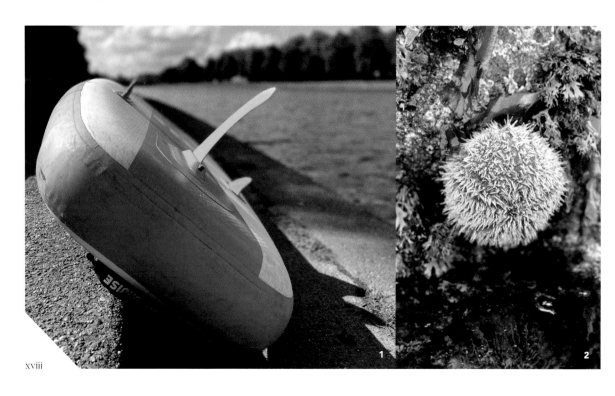

xviii

Safety

GENERAL SAFETY TIPS

» Be fit and healthy enough to paddleboard, including in an emergency.
» Learn about tides, rips, currents, wind and weather. Check forecasts for these before you set out and be aware that conditions may change.
» Always wear a PFD and correct leash.
» If at the coast, do not go out in offshore winds which could blow you out to sea.
» Keep communication equipment like a mobile phone attached to you, not your board.
» Dress for the water temperature, not the air temperature.
» Tell people where you are going, when you are heading out, when you are due back and if you are delayed.
» Complete a SUP training course.
» Watch the online safety videos from British Canoeing, WSA and *SUPfm*.
» Being able to swim confidently will help if and when you fall in.
» Go with a responsible friend so you can help one another should problems arise.

COLD WATER SHOCK

After hearing Professor Mike Tipton speak about cold water shock on Simon Hutchinson's *SUPfm* podcast, I asked him to share with us why we need to dress for the water temperature rather than the air temperature as paddleboarders. He advised that the sudden change from a comfortable air temperature to cold water immersion causes a series of cardiorespiratory responses, including gasping, hyperventilation and panic. Cold shock response includes an increase in heart rate, blood pressure and the work required of the heart; this can even lead to heart attacks.

BIOSECURITY

Invasive non-native species of plants can have a hugely detrimental effect on the waterways we paddle. It is important that as paddlers we don't take invasive species with us. Be sure to check your equipment as you leave the water, clean and wash all equipment and dry equipment and clothing carefully; some species can last for days in moist conditions.

For more information about the impact of invasive species and why we need to be meticulous about Check, Clean and Dry, go to *www.britishcanoeing.org.uk/go-canoeing/access-and-environment/invasive-non-native-species#stop-the-spread*

EMERGENCIES

In an emergency inland, ring **999** and ask for the fire service. In a medical emergency ask for the ambulance service. If you are on an estuary or the coast, ring **999** and ask for the coastguard. Tell them if it is a medical emergency too.

Planning

Creating a plan ahead of your trip not only makes it safer and means you can use your time more effectively, but also adds to the excitement and anticipation. Here are a few things for you to consider when paddling on different bodies of water. The list is not exhaustive, so do check for local conditions.

CANALS

Canals are a great place to start paddle-boarding: they are enclosed, there are lots of places to launch or exit and you will never be far from the towpath. However, they have features to consider.

» **Locks** – paddleboarders don't go through the locks. We leave the canal and carry (or 'portage') our board around the lock.

» **Bridges** – some bridges, for example swing bridges, can be particularly low. If you don't feel comfortable going under them, leave the canal and walk around. Be aware that bridges can funnel the wind.

» **Tunnels** – some longer tunnels require specific permission, so check your route. Some have traffic-light systems, such as Foulridge Tunnel (p191). Paddling on your knees is helpful, as well as fluorescent clothing, torches and a whistle or air horn.

» **Narrowboats** – when approaching oncoming boats, keep to the right-hand side of the canal and pass port to port. Boats may also pass you from behind or create a wash or wake, so if you're unsure just drop to your knees until the water calms down again. Narrowboats have right of way over paddleboards and may not always be able to easily see you.

» **Anglers** – sometimes anglers are tricky to spot if they are hidden behind a bush or tree. Be courteous, let them know that you are there and move to the side to avoid the fishing line.

» **Swans** – move out of their way or leave the canal until they pass.

LAKES, LOCHS AND RESERVOIRS

» **Wind** – large lakes and lochs will be affected by wind which will create waves. Depending on the strength and direction of the wind, returning to shore may be challenging, so check the wind forecast and be prepared for it to change. It may be beneficial to have the wind behind your back on the return journey when you are more tired.

» **Shelter** – paddle close to the edge of the lake/loch/reservoir where it is more sheltered.

» **Outflows and intakes** – be aware of these.

RIVERS

Rivers can be beautiful and they offer the chance to use the river flow to enhance your paddle. If you are new to rivers, start on one that has a gentle, meandering flow.

» **Hazards** – check the water and pollution levels. There is the risk of obstructions from branches, either on or below the surface; your fin may get stuck on rocks or in the mud. Look out for any rapids that are beyond your level of experience or ability.

» **Flow** – a river may be flowing faster beneath the surface. Take into account if it has rained in the days leading up to your paddle as well as the forecast.

» **Weirs** – research how and where to launch and exit safely to go around them.

» **Rowers** – Patricia Carswell, journalist and podcaster at *Girl on the River*, explained that rowers have to stick to a circulation pattern, rowing on the starboard (right-hand) side of the river. Because they face backwards, they can't always see paddleboarders. Wear something luminous to be seen more easily, stay in single file if in a group and do not underestimate how wide their oars are. If you see rowers ahead and you don't think they have seen you, shout 'ahead, rower'.

COASTAL PADDLING

» **Forecast** – learn about the tides and wind. Also check the water quality where you are going.

» **Lifeguards** – paddle from a lifeguarded beach where possible and ask the lifeguards if there is anything you need to know that's unique to the area. A lifeguarded beach will have areas designated for swimmers and bodyboarders only, so avoid these and launch and return between the black-and-white-chequered flags. You can learn the different RNLI flags and what they mean.

» **Coastal erosion** – research this if you are landing on a beach.
» **Estuaries and tidal rivers** – be aware of tides so that you don't find yourself stuck on mudflats. They are hard work to walk across, can be dangerous and you could damage them.

Tips for planning
» **Check the weather and wind forecast.**
» **Check the tides at *www.tidetimes.org.uk* or *www.tide-forecast.com***
» **Check the water quality in the area you are going to using Surfers Against Sewage Safer Seas and Rivers App or the Rivers Trust map.**
» **Other sources to help you plan include *www.riverlevels.uk* and *www.riverapp.net***
» **If you are going somewhere new, researching the area beforehand is important. Look at *www.gopaddling.info* for routes. Get advice from local SUP groups via social media or look for blogs. Do always check the person who is giving the advice knows what they are talking about. Go on a guided tour with a qualified instructor in the area.**
» **Should you fall in a canal, try and stand up. You may be surprised how shallow the water is.**
» **Paddle Logger (for iOS only) uses a GPS that lets you track paddles and add photos. A premium service has features such as sending a text message to friends onshore and a virtual flare in an emergency. RYA SafeTrx, Strava and GeoSUP also allow tracking.**
» **Always be prepared to change your plans according to the conditions on the day.**

ABOVE ALL, REMEMBER 'IF IN DOUBT, DON'T GO OUT.'

Weather

Wind is the primary safety concern when paddleboarding. You should be able to plan, understand and react to the following wind direction and strength and a change in these. Avoid paddling in fog, heavy mist and lightning.

I am grateful to Brendon Prince of The Long Paddle and the water safety charity Above Water for sharing his vast knowledge. His advice is summarised here.

WIND DIRECTION
When commenting on wind direction, observe the direction it is coming from, for example if the wind is coming from the north, it is a northerly wind. To help you understand wind direction, imagine you are standing in the middle of a pie and it's cut into quarters; each quarter represents the wind blowing at you in the middle. The quarter of the pie facing you represents the wind blowing in your face. The quarter pieces to your left and right side are side-on wind and the quarter piece behind you represents tail wind. Wind into your face will dramatically slow your paddling. The chop created by wind from the side will test your balance and ability to paddle in a straight line. The best wind is on your tail or stern. Downwinding will help your paddle speed and make paddling much easier. With all wind directions, the board you paddle on makes a big difference in what can be achieved in each condition.

WIND STRENGTH
For a beginner, a wind speed of only eight kilometres per hour can create uncomfortable paddling conditions. Never go on to the water if the wind is stronger than your ability.

On coastal waters, offshore winds are to be avoided as they have the potential to blow you away from the safety of land. Wind strength will always increase around headlands and further out to sea. If the wind blows above eight kilometres per hour then small waves or a chop will start to develop. If wind has been blowing from the same direction for a long time, over a large stretch of water, then swell will be created. This swell will turn into large waves when it rolls on to a beach or shallow water.

WIND CHANGE
Wind is created by the sun's impact on the sea and land. When the sea is heated by the sun it will suck air off the land, creating an offshore wind or 'land breeze'. You need to understand why local winds occur and how the topography of the coastline can change wind suddenly and affect your paddling.

TIDE HEIGHT
Tide height is the vertical rise or fall of the water through the tidal range. At low tide a muddy and rocky entry or exit may damage your board. At high tide entry or exit may be limited.

TIDAL FLOW OR STREAM
Flow is the movement of water, not the height of the water, and predominantly moves along the beach, NOT in or out.

On a spring tide, the flow of water from left to right or right to left (as you look out to sea) can be two knots (approximately 3.7 kilometres per hour) only 50 metres from the beach. This means you would have to paddle above this speed to feel like you were going in your desired direction. The flow will not carry you into the beach on an incoming tide or out (away from the beach) on an outgoing.

The incoming tide will carry you right to left as you look out to the sea or left to right on an outgoing tide. When flow changes direction you can experience up to one hour of slack water (no flow). As a paddleboarder, slack water can create dangerous currents that will move you in any direction. There are some areas of coastline where the flow is very fast (above five knots) and there can be NO slack time for the water between flow directional change.

Remember spring tides exaggerate the size of high and low tides with greater tidal flow between these extremes. Neap tides create 'middling' conditions: the high tide will not be very high, and the low tide will not be very low. If you are paddling in an area with a large tidal range, like the Severn Estuary (p179), this will increase the tidal flow speeds.

I will often plan my paddle to be with the flow in one direction and then return to my start location with the changing of the tidal flow. Remember tidal flow doesn't always match the times of high or low tides. Find out the tidal flow in your coastal area by checking the Admiralty Tidal Stream Atlas or leading navigation apps.

WIND AGAINST TIDE
For the perfect 'naturally assisted' paddle you need wind on your back and tidal flow in the direction you wish to travel. When wind and flow are against each other the conditions become VERY choppy and paddling is hard work. When wind is against tide, the path of least resistance for your paddle is with the wind – but it's probably going to be a bumpy ride!

Being environmentally thoughtful and responsible

One of the joys of paddleboarding is being able to spend time in nature and the benefits this brings for our physical, mental and emotional well-being. It is important, however, that as paddlers we respect these environments and, where we can, give back to say thank you.

HOW CAN WE MAKE SURE WE PADDLE RESPONSIBLY?

I asked Dr Sarah Perkins, SUPer and Senior Lecturer at Cardiff University's School of Biosciences, about how we can enjoy our time on the water as thoughtfully as possible:

» Watch from a distance and never approach animals: steer a clear course, give lots of space and help them predict your movements. Be careful not to push wildlife along a narrow channel into neighbouring territory where it could be harmed as it defends its home, for example swans. Research where you are going so you know what you might encounter.
» Think about less obvious places that our presence may impact negatively, such as gravel riverbeds where fish spawn, reed beds and sandy areas in the mouth of an estuary.
» Choose carefully when you visit sites to avoid the breeding season from spring to summer and be especially careful not to disturb animals and their young.
» Become a community scientist and conservationist by reporting your plant and animal sightings to iNaturalist. The app will use artificial intelligence to suggest what you have seen, even if you don't know.

SEALS

I was lucky enough to paddle with Charlie Gill, a Marine Stories Ranger from the Cornwall Seal Group Research Trust (p167), who shared some key advice about seals and what we can do to paddle responsibly:

» **Hauling out** – seals need to haul out on land to conduct vital life processes such as pupping, socialising, digesting food and replenishing oxygen levels. When they are hauled out they are incredibly vulnerable to being disturbed.
» **Signs of disturbance** – these include stampeding (when a seal rushes into the sea), tombstoning (when a seal throws itself into the water from a great height), flipper splashing, vocalisation and crash diving, which can all be harmful and even fatal.
» **Reducing your impact** – keep quiet and downwind so seals don't hear or smell you. Be sure to keep a distance of at least 100 metres and do not observe for more than 15 minutes. Also, take your litter home to reduce entanglement and ingestion.
» **Distress** – if you see seals in distress, signal to others and move away quietly. Report the seals you see to *sightings@ cornwallsealgroup.co.uk* who will pass them to the nearest local recording scheme. If you see a seal that you think may need medical attention, phone British Divers Marine Life Rescue on 01825 765546.

DOLPHINS AND WHALES

Keep a distance from dolphins or whales and don't watch them for more than 15 minutes. Do not try to approach, swim with or touch them. For more information, go to *www.ullapoolseasavers.com*

BIRDLIFE

Tony Benton, a wildlife conservationist and birder in West Sussex, explained to me the impact disturbing birds, even unintentionally, can have on their ability to feed and survive. If our approach causes a bird to 'flush' (fly or run away) or change its behaviour we are too close. This might include a change in its posture, freezing, hunching into a protective stance, raising its head or uttering an alarm call.

To be more mindful of birds, paddle quietly and at a distance, kneel down when passing a bird to make your silhouette less threatening and use designated launch points to avoid damaging nesting grounds. Also, carry your board rather than dragging it.

You can read more on the RSPB and BSUPA's Bird Life Paddleboarding Guide, and British Canoeing has a helpful PDF download about birds, whales, seals and dolphins on the access and environment section of its website.

WiSe SCHEME

The WiSe Scheme is an accredited training scheme that provides information for commercial operators in the marine environment to watch wildlife in a wildlife-safe way. As paddleboarders we can also find out more by taking a public module: *www.wisescheme.org*

Making a positive difference to the environment

'I can't change the world, but I can change the little bit around me' is a phrase that's guided me over my paddleboarding journey. With this in mind, there are a number of organisations that are doing incredible work that you can learn from and join:

» Planet Patrol, founded by eco adventurer, environmental campaigner and record-breaking paddleboarder Lizzie Carr MBE, is a global movement of paddleboarders who pick up litter. There are community champions, organised group litter picks and a Planet Patrol app: *www.planetpatrol.co*

» Cal Major has founded both Paddle Against Plastic and the charity Seaful. Seaful's mission is to help more people reconnect to the ocean and waterways, for their mental health and to nurture stewardship of our blue spaces. I am honoured to be an ambassador for Seaful: *www.seaful.org.uk*

» 2 Minute Foundation, founded by writer and environmental campaigner Martin Dorey, is a global community of 'barefoot warriors' encouraged to take just two minutes to pick up litter wherever they are in the world. I am honoured to be an ambassador for it: *www.beachclean.net*

» Clare Osborn, SUP instructor, Blue Health coach and co-founder of #PaddleCleanUp, has written a brilliant download for British Canoeing on how to organise a paddle clean up in your community: *www.britishcanoeing.org.uk*

» Canal & River Trust looks after 3,200 kilometres of waterways in England and Wales. It works towards boosting biodiversity, tackling climate change and invasive species and has its own #PlasticsChallenge campaign. There are lots of ways to volunteer: *www.canalrivertrust.org.uk*

» Surfers Against Sewage is an environmental charity dedicated to protecting the ocean, waves, beaches and wildlife. Founded in 1990 by Cornish surfers, it is led by Hugo Tagholm. It has created the Safer Seas & Rivers Service app and the Million Mile Beach Clean: *www.sas.org.uk*

How I decided which places to include

Choosing which places to share with you has been both wonderful and difficult in equal measure. There are so many beautiful SUP spots and recommendations from paddlers wanting to share the places that are special to them. At times I have been lost in maps and writing research notes.

I have built my list around four key principles:

» **The possibility of place** – I wanted to show the variety of bodies of water we are fortunate enough to have in England, Scotland and Wales. I also wanted to introduce opportunities to view interesting structures from a paddleboard, including lighthouses, sculptures, a crannog, historic buildings, bridges and castles.

» **Range of distance, difficulty and challenges** – this book is aimed at recreational paddleboarders looking for new and interesting places to paddle. There are trips of a kilometre and a half and others of 26 kilometres. My hope is that the variety will offer inspiration to build up to more challenging routes as your experience, skills and knowledge grow. I offer alternatives for those new to paddleboarding and provide details of guided tours so you can enjoy the area with the reassurance of instructors' professional expertise. Your and other people's safety must always be a priority, and a tour would be the best choice if you are in doubt.

I have also chosen places that act as an example to help you understand what you may encounter elsewhere. For example, requiring a licence at Salcombe Harbour (p143) or special permission to paddle through a tunnel.

I have not included SUP racing, SUP surfing or white water SUP, which are distinct disciplines that require expertise, knowledge and specific equipment. I have pointed you to resources where you can learn more.

» **SUP infrastructure** – you will discover places where there are car parks, launch spots and, where possible, public toilets and places to eat. I also include locations that can be reached by rail, bus, metro and tube if you are able to carry your board. I am still working on travelling by bike with a board on my back or finding a good bike trailer – please let me know if you have one! I do not include secret spots or places where an influx of cars parking on the roadside could cause disruption to the local community.

Please remember that many of the coastal areas are seasonal and some shops, cafes and public toilets might not be open outside of the summer. RNLI lifeguards are seasonal too.

» **Balancing exploration SUP spots with honeypots** – honeypots have a detrimental effect on the environment, community and people's experience of their time in the outdoors. I have worked hard to offer alternative ideas and locations not covered in existing SUP guidebooks and online articles. I hope I have struck the right balance in terms of the 'bucket list' and the 'alternative' locations.

Hand on heart, I loved every single place I visited, and in their different ways they inspired me and have enriched my paddleboarding journey. I hope they do for you too.

Reflecting upon my time in Wales, three things stand out clearly: being glued to the wind forecasts, extraordinary wildlife experiences and the SUP family that welcomed me. I began on the River Dee (Afon Dyfrdwy), a magical midsummer evening exploring the river followed by the majestic Llyn Tegid (p23).

A few weeks later, with storms forecast, I set off for West Wales. How lucky we were to get some sunshine. On a paddle with friends along the lush Afon Teifi to Cardigan (p11) we chanced upon friends and witnessed a masterclass in SUP racing.

The blue of the sea along the Ceredigion coastline from Llangrannog to Tresaith will always stay with me (p17). We stood in awe as dolphins swam past and explored a quiet beach.

Oxwich Bay on the Gower peninsula (p5) held its own magic, as we SUP snorkelled from our boards looking for a shipwreck. Rewarded by the sight of a pod of dolphins leaping ahead, we ventured further to the beauty of Three Cliffs Bay.

I squeezed in one final adventure around the Great Orme at Llandudno (p29). The longest sea paddle, requiring the most technical understanding and research, gifted a huge sense of accomplishment.

The beauty of the places I explored and the kindness of the Welsh SUP community outshone the stormy forecasts. These are memories I shall treasure forever.

WALES

Opposite Water lilies on the River Dee, Llyn Tegid **Overleaf** Llyn Tegid (Lake Bala) © Shutterstock/travellight

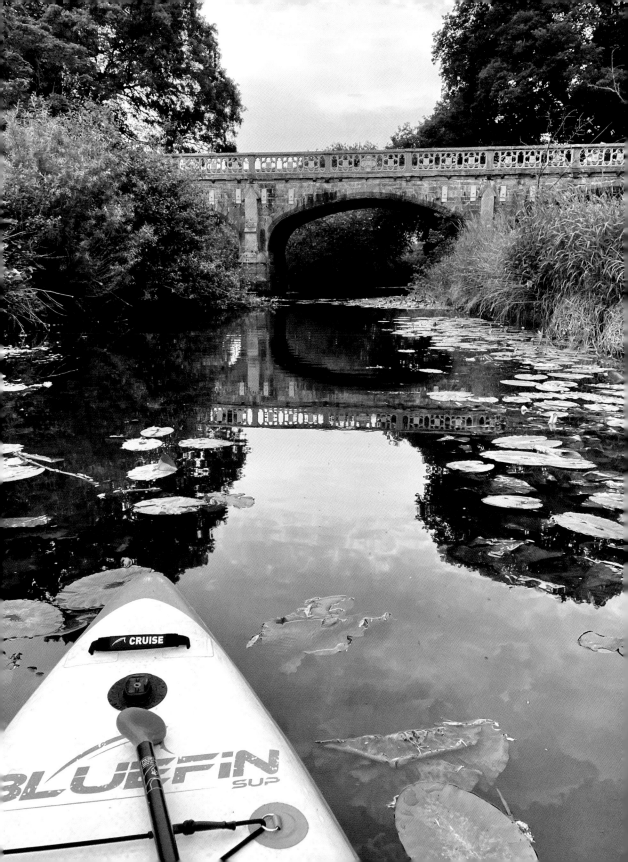

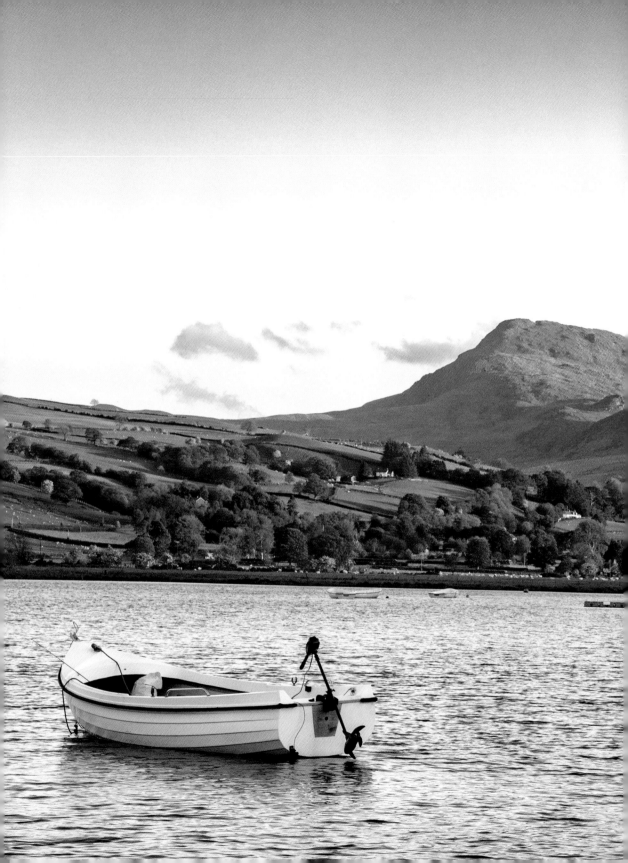

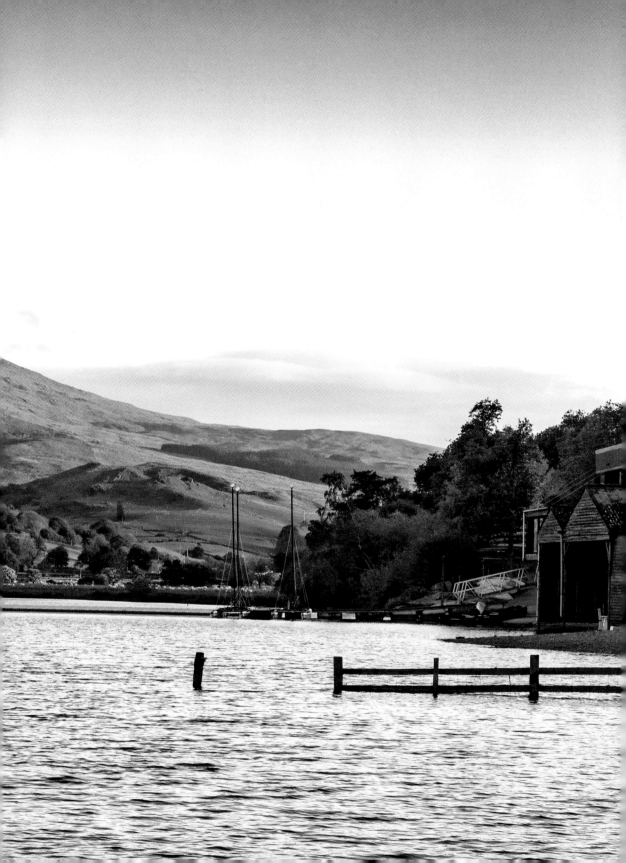

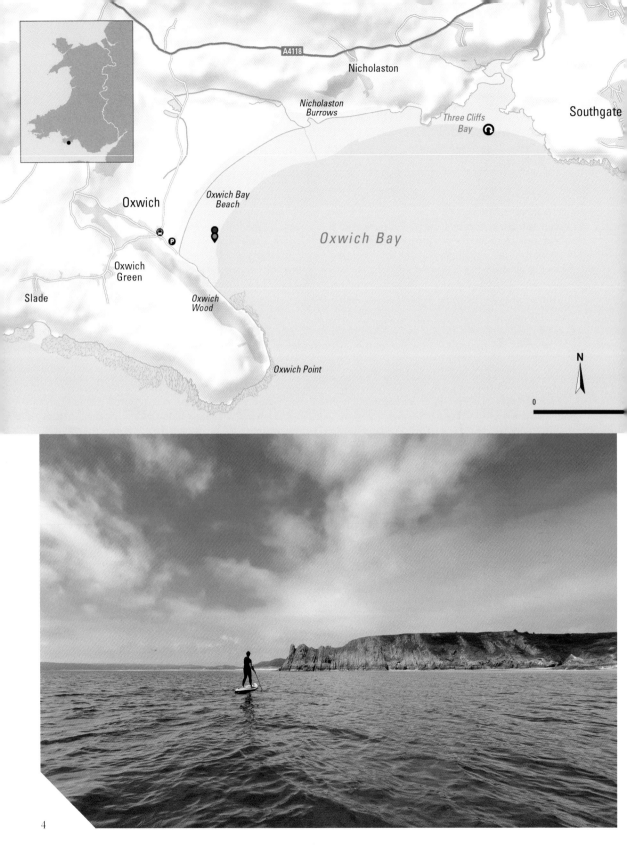

Oxwich

Nicholaston

Nicholaston
Burrows

Three Cliffs
Bay

Southgate

Oxwich Bay
Beach

Oxwich Bay

Oxwich
Green

Slade

Oxwich
Wood

Oxwich Point

N

0

Oxwich Bay

SUP SNORKELLING, A WRECK, DOLPHINS AND PADDLING TO THREE CLIFFS BAY

One of the tiny rituals I have when exploring a new place to SUP is to take a quiet moment to look out at the sea, lake or river and wonder what magic lies ahead. It is no different when I arrive at Oxwich Bay on the south coast of the Gower on a Monday morning, as a glitter path of sunlight sparkles on the water as the waves gently lap the empty beach. I kneel on the sand to breathe in the peace and video the view – a reminder for those wintery months when the days are short and sunshine seems a distant memory. Before I can press record, a car pulls up and a little boy, already in his swimming trunks and rash vest, runs to the water's edge.

'Daddy, daddy,' he squeals, 'the beach is full of water! The sea is here to meet us!' Splashing along the shoreline, his excitement is palpable. He has already discovered the magic of Oxwich Bay and it's not even 9 a.m.

I have come to the Gower to meet Dr Sarah Perkins, Senior Lecturer at Cardiff University's School of Biosciences and also a highly accomplished SUP surfer and racer. We are here not only to paddle on the water but to use our SUPs to explore beneath as well; Sarah has packed a mask and snorkel for me.

Oxwich is a beautiful, golden, four-kilometre-long beach lined with sand dunes and a very gentle slope towards the sea. It sits within the Oxwich National Nature Reserve which also includes lakes, woodlands, cliffs and salt and freshwater marshes further inland. In May and June wild orchids can be seen in the sand dunes, growing in the chalky soil created by crushed shells blown from the beach. The nature reserve is also home to the UK's smallest resident butterfly, the small blue, or (as Sarah

later tells me) *Cupido minimus*. To the east is Nicholaston Burrows (also known as Crawley Beach), then Tor Bay and Three Cliffs Bay. I can see why Oxwich regularly features on 'best beach' lists – the Gower was the first place in Britain to be named an Area of Outstanding Natural Beauty, with its immense sea views, golden sands and dunes.

'We have two options,' says Sarah as we pump up our boards. 'We can have a gentle paddle along the cliff edge, take a look at the wreck and turn back once we reach the outer point of the bay on the west side, or have a longer paddle over to Three Cliffs Bay.' After a busy weekend on the Ceredigion coast in West Wales, a gentle SUP and snorkel sounds perfect. Leaving the beach, we hug the cliff, passing what looks like a fairly significant rockfall, and arrive at a large, white arrow painted on the rock, which marks the point of the wreck of the *Solor*. The *Solor* was a Norwegian vessel torpedoed in the Irish Sea on 27 January 1945 on its way to the Clyde from New York. Two crew members were killed and the ship's hull was badly damaged. Two days later, the *Solor* limped into Oxwich Bay and her cargo was unloaded. The boat soon broke into three, with only the middle section, which is now a popular diving spot, remaining.

We pop on our mask and snorkel, lying diagonally across our boards, and start to explore the world beneath. Our SUPs mean that any boats or jet skis (which are allowed in the bay) as well as other paddlers will be able to see us – they are not simply a platform for our underwater adventures but a safety feature too. Clouds have gathered in the sky and the water visibility is not good, meaning that the wreck and the conger eels Sarah said live within

Opposite Looking back on Oxwich Bay

it remain hidden for today. With a sense of easy companionship we float gently towards a slightly shallower spot and separately explore the rock pools for half an hour, spotting barrel jellyfish and tiny crabs.

Snorkelling is a meditative pastime which requires us to slow our breath and live fully in the moment. I spy a bright-blue plastic shoe wedged between two rocks and spend several minutes pulling it out, along with some plastic wrapping. I'm grateful to have been able to do a tiny #2MinuteBeachClean from my paddleboard.

As we turn back to the beach Sarah spots a pod of common dolphins across the bay, with their distinctive creamy-yellow, hourglass shape on the side. They leap and twist in the air as we stand, mesmerised, for a few minutes, before they continue to swim along the coast. My heart is bursting with joy.

'How do you fancy paddling across to Three Cliffs Bay?' asks Sarah.

'Oh, yes, please,' I reply, energised by the dolphins' visit.

Paddleboarding from the wreck to Three Cliffs Bay takes an hour, and we are met by a stunning beach with the three limestone cliffs, an archway leading to Pobbles Beach and the remains of Pennard Castle on the cliffs above. We watch a horse and rider across the beach and climbers on the rock face. While Oxwich Bay Beach is not lifeguarded, Three Cliffs Bay is in the summer months as there are strong rip currents and tidal systems. For more about rip currents do read William Thomson's *The Book of Tides* and Tristan Gooley's *How to Read Water*.

We set off back to Oxwich Bay Beach, and with the sea breeze it takes around two hours to reach. We also need to walk for a few minutes from the shoreline to our cars as the tide is now

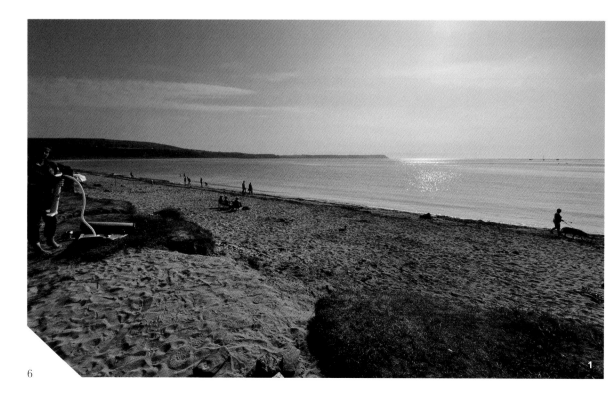

1

1 Pumping up our boards at Oxwich Bay Beach 2 Sarah enjoying our magical paddle

going out. Stopping to look at starfish (or sea stars) and sea potatoes on the way, we take a moment to listen to the mud 'singing' as the water drains through.

A few days later I read an article by Stuart Gammon in *Stand Up Paddle Mag UK* about a trip starting inland at the Gower Heritage Centre, going along the Pennard Pill and arriving at Three Cliffs beach. Another friend messages me about her evening paddle with Stuart down the river. Adventures for another day.

From the gentle SUP snorkel to the more demanding paddle to Three Cliffs Bay, Oxwich Bay has gifted us a day of wonder and curiosity. As the little boy splashing in the waves had expressed so accurately earlier in the day, the sea came up to meet us and shared a very special kind of salty magic. I hope you'll experience it too.

Technical information

> DISTANCE
> TO THE WRECK **2km round trip.**
> TO THREE CLIFFS BAY **9km round trip.**
> ....
> LAUNCH LOCATION
> ENTRY AND EXIT POINT **SS 506864/51.556, -4.158**
> TURN AROUND POINT **SS 536875/51.566, -4.113**
> ....
> ALTERNATIVE ROUTE **Paddling to Three Cliffs Bay is more demanding due to it being windier and more exposed than the paddle to the wreck, so spending your time on the water close to the beach would be lovely.**

Difficulty

An understanding of wind and tides is important when paddleboarding on the sea. Oxwich Bay is well protected from the prevailing southwesterly wind and only gets waves when there is a large swell running. A northerly wind

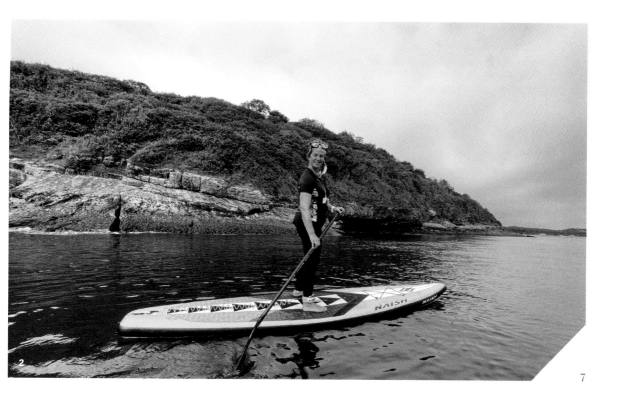

here is dangerous and will send you straight out to sea. Be careful heading along the west shore on an outgoing tide, as the tide can flow very quickly out of the bay, especially at Oxwich Point. It is best to time a paddle to the wreck on an incoming tide.

Getting there

There is a bus from Swansea to Nicholaston Cross and then a 4km walk to the launch point. Buses from Horton also stop just outside the Dunes Cafe and Shop. The nearest railway stations are Swansea and Gowerton.

Oxwich Bay is about 22.5km by car from Swansea. Once you reach the Dunes Cafe and Shop in Oxwich, turn left towards the beach. You will soon come to a large, paid car park (SS 502864/51.557, -4.162), where there are public toilets. Recent restrictions have been put in place regarding where motorhomes and campervans can park; follow the instructions provided.

Route information

Be aware the tide goes out a long way, so you may have longer to walk and less to paddle.

There are no lifeguards at Oxwich Bay Beach, but there are in the summer months at Three Cliffs Bay.

There is also no webcam, but GowerLive has webcams on several beaches along the Gower.

Eating and drinking

» There are a couple of food kiosks by the beach, or alternatively you could bring a picnic or stock up at Oxwich's Village Shop.
» The Oxwich Bay Hotel is close to the beach.
» The award-winning, Michelin-starred Beach House Restaurant is very close to the beach.

Instruction, guided tours and equipment hire

» Stuart Gammon of SUPDude.Stu runs river paddles and after-dark glow paddles at Three Cliffs Bay, as well as sunset SUP at Rhossili Bay. He also offers beginner, intermediate and one-on-one lessons.
» Oxwich Watersports offers paddleboard hire.

Further information

Natural Resources Wales provides information on Oxwich National Nature Reserve: *www.naturalresources.wales*

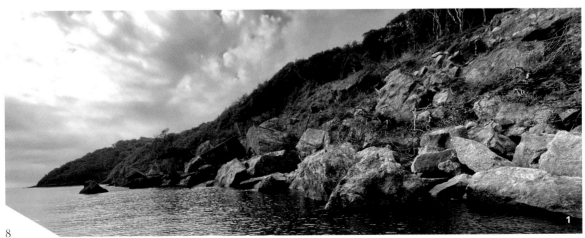

1

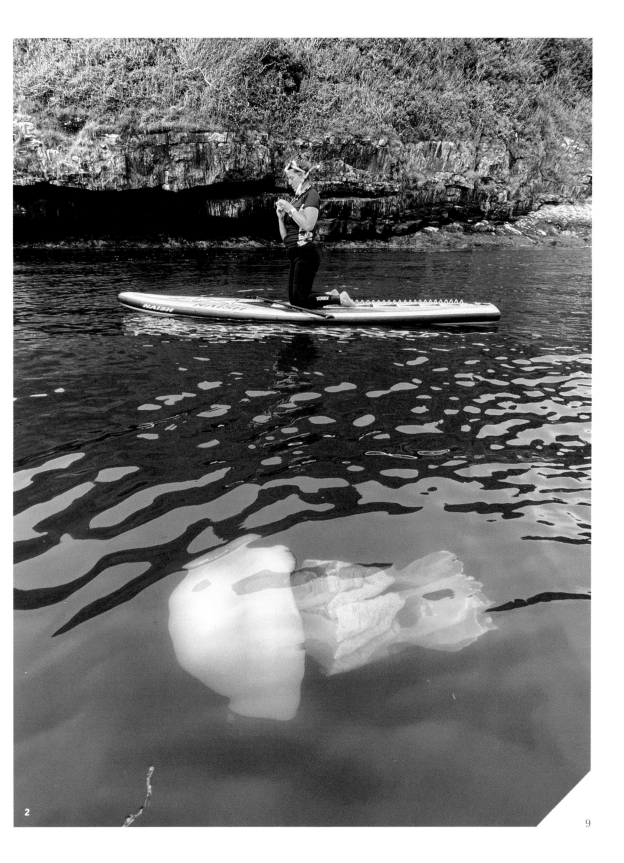

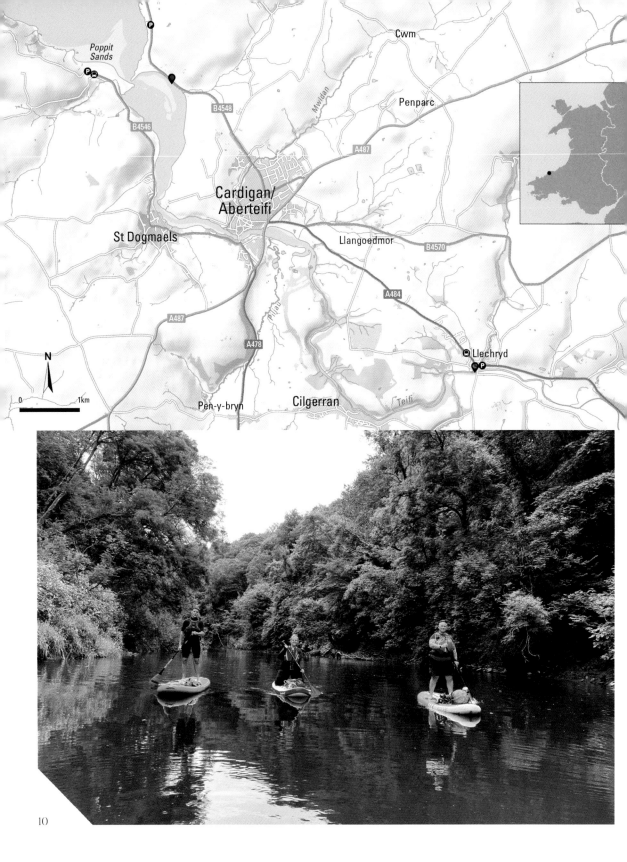

Afon Teifi

LUSH, GREEN WOODLAND, RED KITES, RAPIDS AND A CASTLE

Thunderstorms and weather warnings. This is the forecast for the weekend I plan to be in West Wales to paddle along the Afon Teifi and Ceredigion coastline.

'I'm continuing to keep an eye on the weather, wind and swell,' messages Clare Rutter, Canoe Wales's first, and at the time only, #ShePaddles Ambassador. 'Conditions are improving!' comes her text one day. 'You will still need your cagoule though,' she adds. Like many of us in the UK, I've often paddleboarded in the rain. As long as it's safe, I'm always happy to bring my own 'internal' sunshine. I pack my waterproofs and sunscreen and remain hopeful.

Having travelled from Yorkshire through the stunning Cambrian Mountains and Aberaeron, with its pretty, brightly coloured houses, I am keen to stretch my legs. After a beautiful sunset walk at Aberporth, watching teenagers laughing and playing on their paddleboards in the bay, we check the forecast for the Afon Teifi before bed – maybe, just maybe, we won't need our cagoules.

At 122 kilometres, the Afon Teifi is one of the longest rivers entirely in Wales. Along with the tributaries, most of the river is designated a Special Area of Conservation. Rising in the remote Teifi Pools in the Cambrian Mountains, it passes through wetlands and farmland, through the Teifi Gorge, the Teifi Marshes Nature Reserve and on to the castle and quay in Cardigan and the estuary leading to Poppit Sands. The river is tidal in the lower stretch after Llechryd, which is something to take into account when planning your trip, and there is the chance of some small rapids to navigate too.

To help with logistics, we leave one car at Patch Beach where we will later exit, then drive to Llechryd village to park down the lane by the bridge. This stretch of the riverbank is owned by Jet Moore of Adventure Beyond, where Clare is a SUP instructor. Jet is happy to allow access from the slipway or bank on the left-hand side of the river looking downstream; a donation to Save Our Rivers would be appreciated in return.

Along with Lucy and Lisa, friends from the local Facebook paddleboarding community, we launch here on to a lush stretch of river flanked by woodland. Lisa points out ash, beech, hazel, sycamore and willow trees, and we hear and spot red kites above. Paddling and chatting side by side, Lisa shares a lovely conservation story about them: after numbers dwindled almost to extinction in Wales, rural communities, dedicated volunteers and organisations such as the Welsh Kite Trust came together to protect these magnificent birds. According to the RSPB, Wales now has over 400 pairs.

I notice the banks of the river are covered with slate, a reminder of the historical quarrying in the area that once employed hundreds of people and ended in 1938. Debris from the quarries filled the river so much that larger boats were no longer able to navigate it.

We soon arrive at Cilgerran, where by chance we meet SUP racing champion and head coach of Swansea SUP Club Emily King, who is holding a paddleboarding masterclass. We stand on the grassy bank and watch in awe of her technique, speed and skill. The Welsh paddleboarding community feels very warm and welcoming. Enjoying our tea and cake, I learn about coracles, traditional oval, flat-bottomed boats made from willow and hazel. A number of fishermen are licensed to fish for salmon, trout and 'sewin' (sea trout) here in

Opposite Lucy, Lisa and Clare on the Afon Teifi

11

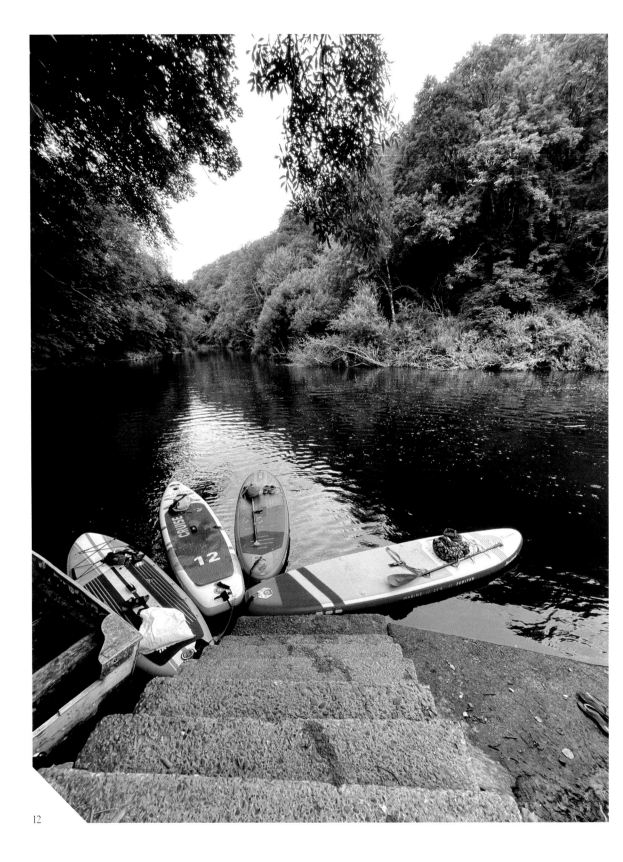

coracles and there are races at Cenarth and Cilgerran at village festivals in the summer. If you have time, Cilgerran Castle is a few minutes' walk from the village, as is Siop Y Pentre, the local village post office and refill shop which Lisa tells me sells great coffee.

Back on the water, we head through the Teifi Gorge, where the banks are much steeper, and keeping to the left we paddle through the grade I rapids with lots of laughter and delight. There are families swimming in the river and I take a quiet moment to pause and soak up the dappled sunlight. Next is the Teifi Marshes Nature Reserve, where we leave the river and walk up to the Welsh Wildlife Centre for lunch at the beautiful Glasshouse Cafe. I spot a whiteboard in the visitor centre with a list of the birds and wildlife that have been seen in the last month, with deer, kingfishers, otters, curlews, newts and grass snakes among them.

There is another small rapid as we head towards Cardigan and this time I take off my main fin to make a smoother ride, watched over by swans and Canada geese. At this point the river widens and, depending on the tide, can get a little muddy. We pass under a bridge and then stop at Adventure Beyond's office and chat to Jason Wilkins, woodturner and owner of Old Forge Crafts which displays his beautiful work. At the next bridge we arrive at Cardigan Castle. The castle is believed to be the birthplace of

Wales's biggest cultural festival, the Eisteddfod, in 1176. Salmon swim towards us as we take a moment by the Cardigan Bridge, which was built in 1247. At every point, there is something to learn.

The estuary continues to widen as we paddle past boats – being sure to keep clear of stern and bow lines – and bear right, passing St Dogmaels. The river then straightens and there are two exit points you might consider, depending on the tide and your energy levels: one is at the Ferry Inn, where there is a pontoon, and the other is the 'mermaid slipway', a slipway with a lovely mermaid statue beside it. We have another stretch to go to reach the car at Patch Beach, making it a paddle of almost 11 kilometres, although with the river flow it didn't feel demanding.

Before we head home, Clare takes me to Gwbert viewpoint so we can see where the lower Teifi Estuary meets the waters of Cardigan Bay and where our journey ultimately ends. It is a stunning view along the coastline and a perfect way to reflect upon a day of community, conservation stories and the history of this beautiful part of West Wales. I would definitely add this to your paddle if you can. Despite the weather warnings earlier in the week, the sun most definitely shone on our world that day, literally and metaphorically. I do hope it does for you too.

Opposite Leaving our boards for a snack at Cilgerran

Technical information

DISTANCE **11km one way.**

LAUNCH LOCATION
ENTRY POINT **SN 218436/52.062, -4.601**
EXIT POINT **SN 166483/52.102, -4.679**

ALTERNATIVE ROUTE **You could break up the journey and launch at different points along the river. With a car, launch at Cilgerran where there is a car park, toilets and the nearby shop Siop Y Pentre.**

Difficulty

Paddleboarding on rivers takes planning, thought and an understanding of the obstacles and the equipment required.

There are grade I rapids on this route.

Getting there

The nearest railway station is Aberystwyth, and from here there are regular buses to Cardigan. Buses between Carmarthen and Cardigan stop 300m from the launch point. Buses to Cardigan also stop by the Poppit Sands Beach car park.

If you park at Llechryd (SN 218437/52.063, -4.601), park near the bridge, not the hotel track, and please do make a donation to Save Our Rivers.

Eating and drinking

» Siop Y Pentre local village shop and post office, where you can buy sandwiches, snacks and hot drinks.
» We had a lovely lunch at the Glasshouse Cafe at the Welsh Wildlife Centre near Cardigan.
» Jason Wilkins, owner of Old Forge Crafts, sells snacks and drinks from his charming shop in Cardigan located on The Strand, just a few hundred metres from the river.

Instruction, guided tours and equipment hire

» Adventure Beyond runs guided tours on the Afon Teifi and the coast near Cardigan. The owner, Jet Moore, owns the stretch of riverbank where we parked at Llechryd.
» Leanne Bird Wellbeing & Adventure offers SUP lessons, coaching and SUP yoga around Cilgerran.
» Dennis Stanfield of SUP Cilgerran.

Further information

» Find out more about Emily King, her masterclasses and adventures: *www.emilykingpaddle.co.uk*
» The Welsh Kite Trust: *www.welshkitetrust.wales*

1 A peaceful moment at the Welsh Wildlife Centre **2** Paddling in Cardigan **3** Clare paddling near Cardigan Castle **4** Aberporth **5** Our launch location at Llechryd **6** Looking out to the estuary near Patch Beach, where we parked

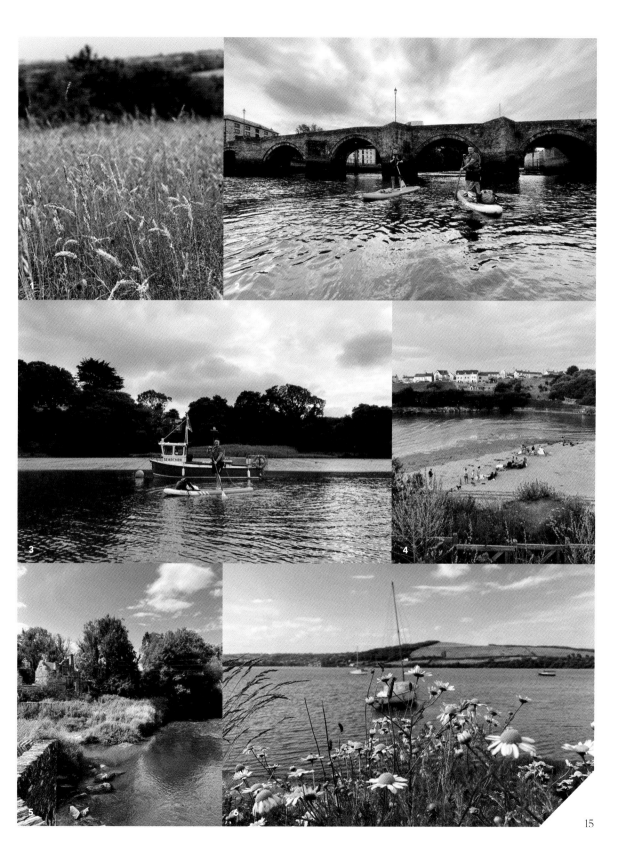

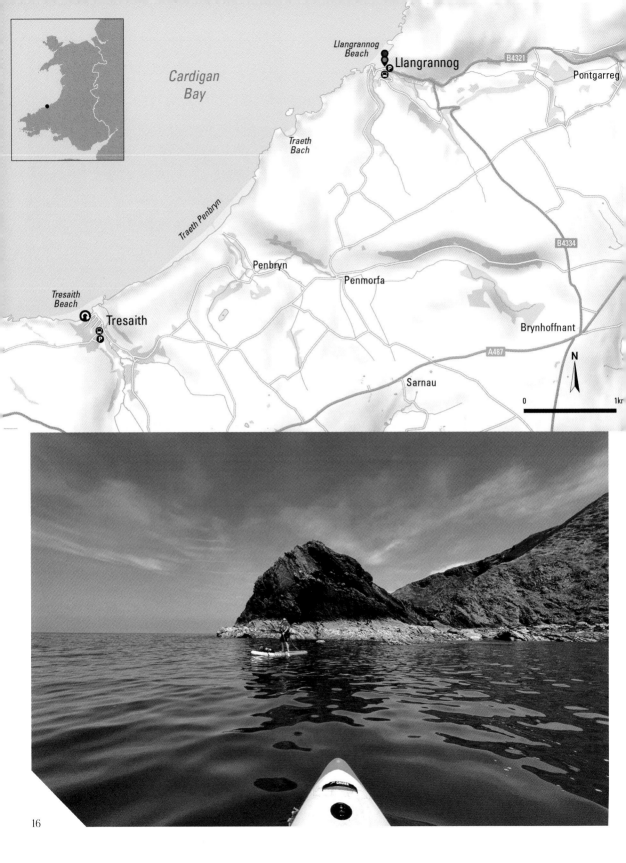

Llangrannog to Tresaith

DOLPHINS, MAGNIFICENT JELLYFISH, QUIET BEACHES AND A DIP IN THE SEA

'Wow, it's huge!' I gasp, kneeling on my paddleboard to get a closer view of the barrel jellyfish floating close by. With their mushroom-shaped head, eight frilly tentacles and violet fringe, barrel jellyfish can grow up to 90 centimetres across and weigh 35 kilograms. I am in awe watching it in the turquoise waters off the Ceredigion coast, and make a note to learn more about them when I'm home.

Curiosity and learning about a landscape and its wildlife have played an important part in my paddleboarding joy over the years. Finding wonder in the tiniest of details not only adds to the moment but also creates a sense of belonging, if only briefly, to new spots. Memories feel more intimate; I have experienced rather than simply visited a place.

'Dolphins, there are dolphins,' whispers Sarah while pointing to a small pod swimming past, their dorsal fins sparkling in the sunshine as they dive and surface before us. First the jellyfish, now the dolphins – I can't help bursting into tears.

Sarah, Clare (Canoe Wales #ShePaddles Ambassador) and I have set out on a coastal adventure in West Wales, the day after Clare and I paddled the Afon Teifi from Llechryd to Cardigan (p11). Thankfully, the weather warnings of thunderstorms forecast for the weekend have not materialised and we awoke to clear skies. Our plan is to SUP from Llangrannog to Tresaith and back, taking in these two beautiful beaches along the Ceredigion coastline, part of the Wales Coast Path. It will be a round trip of nearly nine kilometres. The Wales Coast Path is the first path in the world that follows the country's coastline in its entirety, and a friend,

Zoe Langley-Wathen, was the first woman to walk the 1,400-kilometre route in 2012.

Our launch point, Llangrannog, is a small seaside village lying within the steep-sided valley of the Nant Hawen. The main beach, known as Traeth y Pentref or the Village Beach, lies beneath craggy cliffs. On the north side of the shore is an unusually shaped rock named Carreg Bica, which according to legend was once a giant's tooth that he spat out after suffering from toothache. At low tide you can walk around the rock to the more hidden Cilborth Cove.

We arrive in Llangrannog early enough to secure a parking spot at the car park a few steps away from the beach. The beach, which is pebbly close to the village but then becomes sandy closer to the water, is already filling up, and it has a friendly, family-orientated feel about it.

We make sure to launch away from swimmers and children playing in the sea. As we head south out of the bay, blue skies with just a touch of cloud and a beautiful view of the coastline greet us. There is barely a breeze, the sea is calm and sunlight dances on the water. We paddle along, sometimes chatting, sometimes lost in our own thoughts. Nothing is hurried, there is nowhere to be other than exactly where we are.

We soon arrive at Traeth Bach or Little Beach, a secluded, sandy cove with high cliffs. We pull our boards out of the water on the north side, Carreg-y-Ty, where there is a small sea cave, and take a moment to sit in the sun. We will be back for a swim later.

Opposite Pointing towards Llangrannog

The next stop is the National Trust's kilometre-and-a-half-long Penbryn Beach. There is a woodland behind the beach, full of wood anemones in the spring, as well as a car park around 450 metres away, public toilets and The Plwmp Tart cafe – a launch point for another day, perhaps.

A couple of hours after leaving Llangrannog we reach Tresaith, with the Afon Saith waterfall marking the entrance. It is a bustling beach, and like Llangrannog has RNLI lifeguards, public toilets and places to eat. It's time for lunch! Clare has brought a padlock, meaning we can safely tie the three boards up and head to The Ship Inn, passing a very long queue for Siop y Traeth, which sells Mary's Farmhouse ice cream. Equally busy is the Tresaith Beach Grill, a pretty, blue Airstream serving drinks, breakfast and burgers. By a stroke of luck, there is a table for us at The Ship Inn and we enjoy a chilled lunch with a view of the sea, bringing our paddles and safety kit with us to the pub.

It's time for us to head back to Traeth Bach for a dip. The cliffs along the coast rise high above and we quietly watch a particular oystercatcher perched on a ledge. A couple of snorkellers are exploring the cove and there are hikers and people relaxing, eating picnics and reading. We paddle carefully on to Carreg-y-Ty through the rocky outcrop, with just enough waves to feel like water explorers, and carry our boards on to the beach. Ready for a peaceful dip, we are grateful for the opportunity to both SUP and swim in the warm, clear waters. It's a bit of a trek on foot to reach Traeth Bach, but on our boards it has been a joyful paddle along the coast.

Another jellyfish catches our eye out at sea, this time a lion's mane, with its long and very stingy tentacles. We keep a distance, glad to study it from the safety of our SUPs. The tide is out as we arrive back at Llangrannog, but it is just a couple of minutes to the car park. With everything safely packed away it is time to explore the village. I'm excited to see a #2MinuteBeachClean board being put to good use.

Enjoying a nice cup of tea and sharing a piece of Guinness cake from Tafell a Tân, winner of Best Street Food in Wales Award 2018,

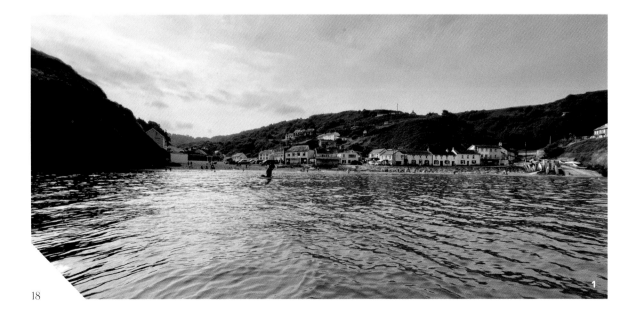

we reflect upon our watery adventure: sunshine, friendship, dolphins, jellyfish and a dip in the turquoise sea. For a perfect summer spot with moments of awe and wonder, Llangrannog to Tresaith has been ideal. I would return in a heartbeat. I hope you will visit too.

Technical information

DISTANCE **8.8km round trip.**

....

LAUNCH LOCATION
ENTRY AND EXIT POINT **SN 311542/52.160, -4.471**
TURN AROUND POINT **SN 278515/52.135, -4.518**

....

ALTERNATIVE ROUTE **You could paddle from Llan-grannog to Tresaith and take the bus or a taxi back or vice versa.**

Difficulty

Paddleboarding experience is necessary for this trip and knowledge of wind and tides is important for Llangrannog to Tresaith. Paddleboarding close to the beaches in the enclosed bay would be a lovely alternative.

Getting there

Llangrannog

The nearest railway station to Llangrannog is Carmarthen, approximately 44km away. Infrequent buses to Cardigan stop in the village, and also stop in Tresaith.

There is a pay-and-display car park just by Llangrannog's beach (SN 311542/52.160, -4.470), and also a free car park at the top of the village if you are happy to carry your board down. There are public toilets in the village.

Tresaith

You can reach Tresaith from Cardigan via an infrequent bus.

There is a car park at the top of a steep hill (SN 279513/52.133, -4.515), around 300m from the beach.

Route information

Both Llangrannog and Tresaith's beaches are lifeguarded during the summer. There is a webcam at the Pentre Arms of Llangrannog Beach.

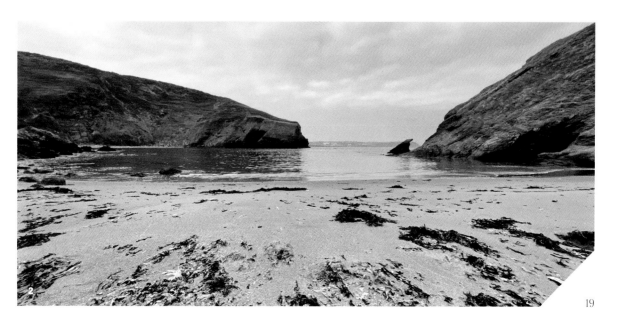

1 Sarah paddling a few minutes after leaving Llangrannog   **2** Traeth Bach
3 Compass jellyfish   **4** Leaving Llangrannog   **Opposite** Approaching Tresaith

Eating and drinking

Llangrannog

» We had a cup of tea and cake at Tafell
a Tân. It also sells award-winning pizzas.
» There were huge queues of ice cream fans
at Caffi Patio, which makes homemade
ice cream.

Tresaith

» We had a lovely lunch at The Ship Inn.
» The Tresaith Beach Grill had a great-
looking menu.

Instruction, guided tours and equipment hire

Llangrannog

» Caiacs Carreg Bica Kayaks.

Tresaith

» The Beach Shop rents kayaks and it has
a limited number of paddleboards.

Further information

» Zoe Langley-Wathen:
www.headrightout.com
» Alistair Hare, *The Beaches of Wales: The
complete guide to every beach and cove
around the Welsh coastline* (Vertebrate
Publishing, 2020).
» Susanne Masters, *Wild Waters: A wildlife
and water lover's companion to the aquatic
world* (Vertebrate Publishing, 2021).

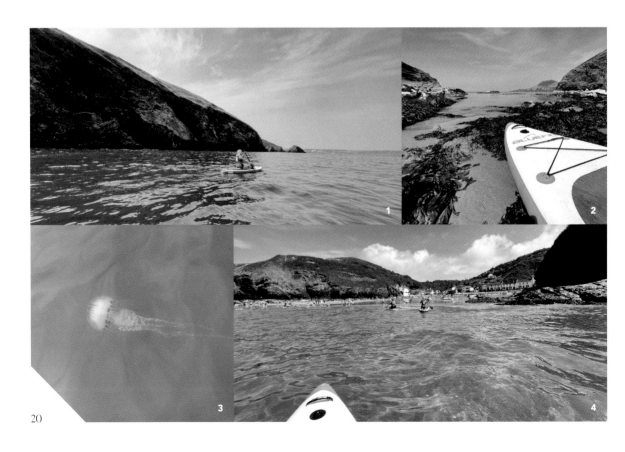

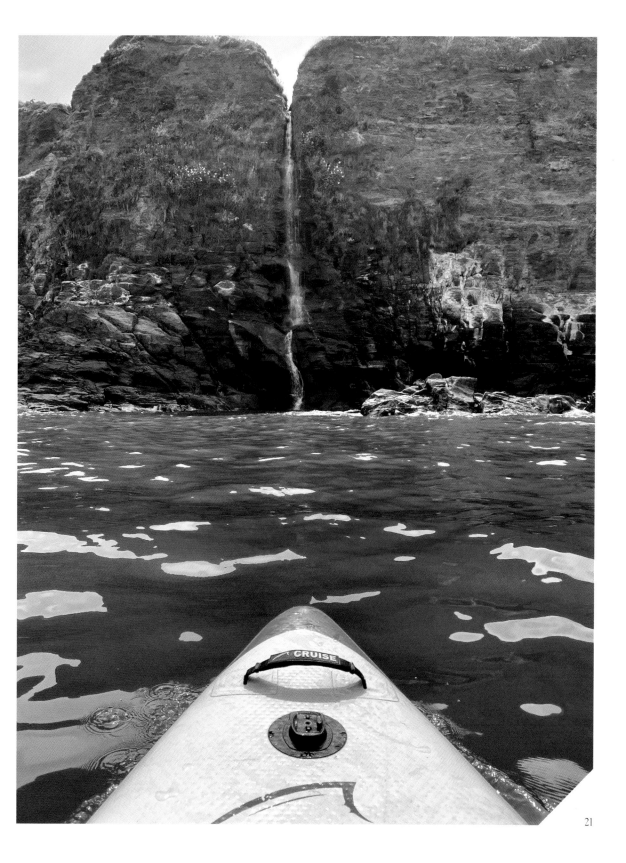

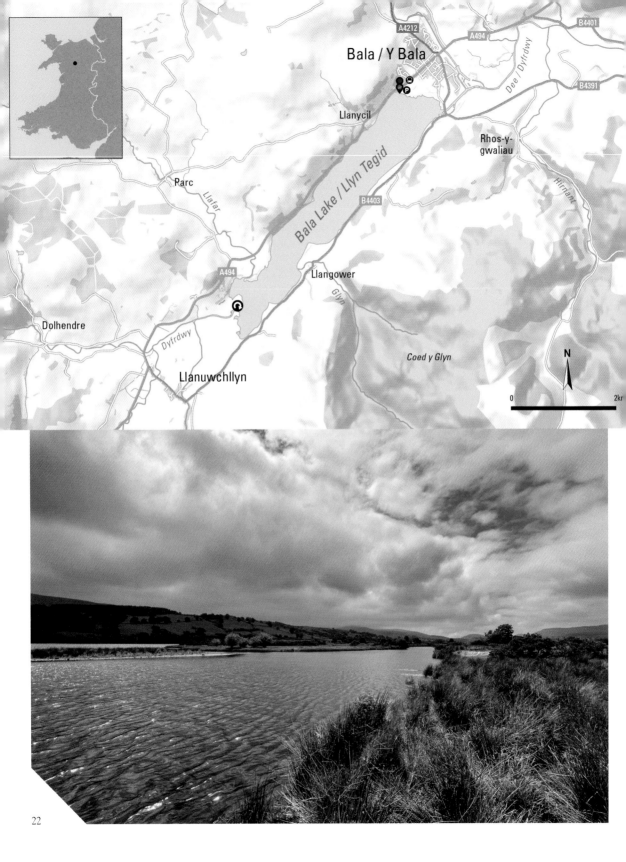

Llyn Tegid (Lake Bala)

MIDSUMMER DREAMS ON THE RIVER DEE (AFON DYFRDWY)

'It's magical, like *A Midsummer Night's Dream*,' I say, looking at the beautiful, blue bridge, the pink sunset and water lilies around my board. We have paddled along a small creek leading from the River Dee (Afon Dyfrdwy). For a moment, it feels like we've stepped into another world. If it were not for the mosquitoes tucking into my legs, I could have stayed for hours soaking up this enchanted spot.

It is almost 10 p.m. and I am paddling with Caroline (Caz) Dawson, founder of SUP Lass Paddle Adventures who I first came across on Simon Hutchinson's paddleboarding podcast *SUPfm*, and her partner Jonathan along the River Dee. They have kindly invited me to stay with them before we research Llyn Tegid, also known as Bala Lake, in the eastern edge of Snowdonia National Park. Taking the opportunity to enjoy the longest Saturday of the year, we have paddled to the beautiful Aldford Iron Bridge, linking the village of Aldford with the Duke of Westminster's Eaton Hall estate. During the day, this stretch is often busy with other paddlers, rowers and canoeists, but for now it is just us, carefully watching for the deer that Caroline sometimes spots. Choosing to paddle at a time when everyone else is tucked up in bed really can gift a special and different experience.

'Gosh, I'm normally asleep by now,' I joke as we gently paddle back to the launch point, and Caz gives me a feather as a souvenir of our trip. 'But this is so beautiful, I'm grateful you shared it with me,' I add.

After Jonathan's delicious breakfast the next day, we travel to Bala, a historic market town at the head of Llyn Tegid in south Snowdonia, to meet Clare Rutter, a SUP instructor and #ShePaddles Ambassador for Canoe Wales. I have also been fortunate to paddle with Clare along the Afon Teifi and Ceredigion coastline (p11). We park close to the edge of the lake and I lean forward – the view is simply breathtaking. It is a grey, overcast day but I can see the mountains rising majestically in the distance.

Llyn Tegid is the largest freshwater glacial lake in Wales at approximately six kilometres long, just under a kilometre wide and 42 metres deep. Bala means the outlet point of a lake, and the River Dee flows in at the southern end and out at the northern, where the town is located. According to local legend, the lake is named after Tegid Foel, a character from early native Welsh tales and husband of the enchantress Ceridwen.

Llyn Tegid is part of British Canoeing's Three Lakes Challenge. With Loch Awe in Scotland and Windermere in the Lake District, the challenge is to paddle the length of all three in the fastest time possible. In June 2021, David Haze achieved a world record as the first person to paddle these three, plus Lough Neagh in Northern Ireland, in the fastest time, all while fundraising for a charity that uses sport and physical activity in the criminal justice system.

The lake is surrounded by three mountain ranges – Aran, Arenig and Berwyn – which all formed around 500 million years ago. The lake is a Site of Special Scientific Interest and Ramsar wetlands a site of international importance. Teeming with birdlife and wildlife, it is a nature lover's delight. It is also home to the gwyniad, a whitefish which is found only in Llyn Tegid. Despite our best efforts, however, we don't spot it, nor the fabled Teggie monster.

Access is easy as we simply walk into the water; although there is a pontoon,

Opposite Looking out on Llyn Tegid

1 Jonathan, Caz and Clare on Llyn Tegid **2** Approaching the spit of land where sheep are grazing

only customers of Bala Adventures and Watersports can use it. There are swimmers, kayakers and families with paddleboards hired from the water sports centre having fun. We paddle on the north-western side of the lake not far from the shoreline, watching for branches and rocks, and pass a couple of anglers. Within just a few minutes we are the only paddleboarders making our way down the lake, and it feels like we are on a wild adventure.

The gentle breeze we felt at the shore has started to strengthen and we soon find ourselves being pushed along by the wind. 'Yay, a bit of downwinding!' says Caz enthusiastically.

'Hmmm ...' I reply cautiously. I'll be honest, I am a little more comfortable paddling into the wind than being pushed by it. After a few minutes, I decide to kneel and enjoy watching the others confidently fly across the water.

Under Caz's guidance we keep an eye out for the posts and spit of land that sticks out about three quarters of the way down the lake. Sheep are grazing in the fields close to the water and the mountain range in the distance looks magnificent.

We are soon close to the end of the lake and it is time for a cup of tea and cake. Caz has brought her trusty Kelly Kettle and we enjoy a brew and sticky ginger cake with an extraordinarily beautiful view of the lake and Aran mountains. It is wonderful to think the River Dee flows into the lake, and while our paddling spot of last night is 66 kilometres away the two are connected by a tapestry of waterways.

Back on the water we begin our return paddle, chatting about our adventures to come. We pass the beach and campsite of

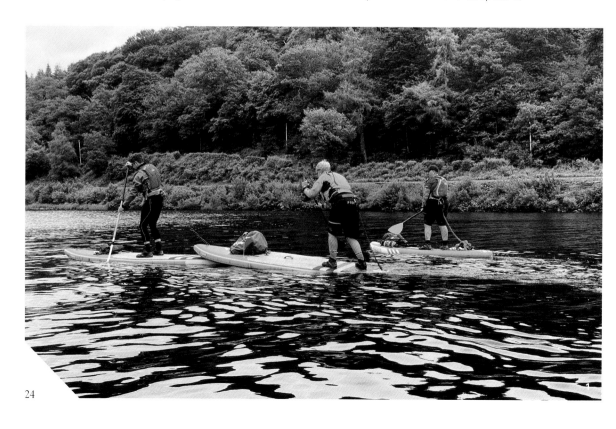

Pant Yr Onnen and I spy a couple of shepherd's huts. How relaxing would it be to wake up on the edge of the lake with a day of swimming and SUP ahead? Maybe next year. Further on, we hear Alice the Little Welsh Engine, running alongside the lake from Llanuwchllyn to Bala. The gorgeous red train is a lovely sight and adds to the charm of our day's paddling.

Arriving back at the shore, after just over 10.5 kilometres, we see two young girls of perhaps 12 or 13 years old playing on their boards, laughing and jumping in the water. Caz compliments their skills and then encourages them to try a step back turn (stepping back on your board so the end sinks into the water and allows you to pivot quickly). One of the girls cautiously, but with determination, tries and successfully turns her board. I watch as her face lights up and her friend looks on, glowing with pride. This is a tiny moment and yet such a powerful one – I hope they will remember this afternoon of confidence on the water. Paddleboarding is still a relatively young sport and encouraging each other today is part of the community we are creating for tomorrow. It is the perfect end to a wonderful adventure.

With a stop at Aran Hufen lâ Ice Cream for a delicious carrot cake ice cream, we are on our way home after a day of lakes and mountains in Snowdonia. *Diolch yn fawr iawn,* Caz, Clare and Jonathan. This has been my first weekend paddleboarding in Wales and it has been extraordinary. A midsummer weekend of enchanted paddling, big views and tea by the lake. I hope one day you'll get to experience this magic too.

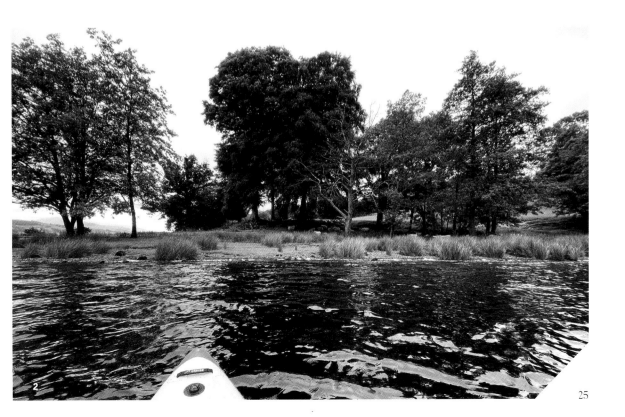

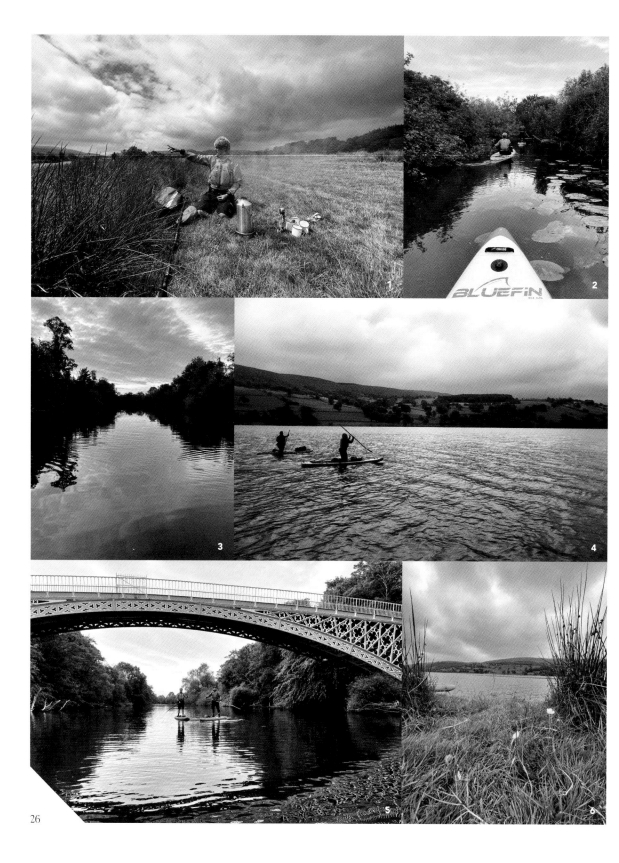

Technical information

DISTANCE **10.6km round trip.**

LAUNCH LOCATION
ENTRY AND EXIT POINT **SH 921355/52.906, -3.606**
TURN AROUND POINT **SH 890315/52.869, -3.651**

Difficulty
Paddleboarding the length of the lake requires an understanding of wind conditions and obstacles along the shoreline. Paddling close to the beach area is a lovely alternative on a calm day.

Getting there
The nearest railway station is Blaenau Ffestiniog, 33km away. A bus from Barmouth to Wrexham stops in Bala, 300m from the launch point.

There is a pay-and-display car park right on the shoreline of Llyn Tegid (SH 921355/52.906, -3.605).

Route information
You need to buy a launch permit to paddle on Llyn Tegid. This can be bought by the Foreshore car park pay and display, and is payable to Snowdonia National Park.

Snowdonia National Park has a webcam overlooking Llyn Tegid, updated every five minutes.

Other than safety boats, power boats and sailing crafts longer than 5.8m are not allowed on the lake.

Eating and drinking
» We visited the handmade ice cream shop, Aran Hufen Iâ, on the High Street in Bala.
» The seasonal Lakeview Cafe at Bala Sailing Club is open to the public.

Instruction, guided tours and equipment hire
» Caroline Dawson, founder of SUP Lass Paddle Adventures, offers beginner lessons and tuition, guided tours, coastal journey and adventure planning as well as SUP socials.
» You can hire boards from Bala Adventure and Watersports, including large and extra-large boards for up to six people. You are required to stay within a limited distance of the shore.
» Tony Bain, owner of Green Dragon Activities based on Bala's High Street, runs beginner and improver classes, guided tours, board hire and paddleboard sales.

Further information
» Alice the Little Welsh Engine, Bala Lake Railway: *www.bala-lake-railway.co.uk*
» British Canoeing's Three Lakes Challenge: *www.britishcanoeing.org.uk*

1 Time for tea and cake at the side of Llyn Tegid   **2** The lush River Dee   **3** The River Dee at sunset   **4** Kneeling as we are pushed along by the wind © Caroline Dawson (SUP Lass Paddle Adventures)   **5** The beautiful Aldford Iron Bridge on the River Dee   **6** A glimpse of Llyn Tegid

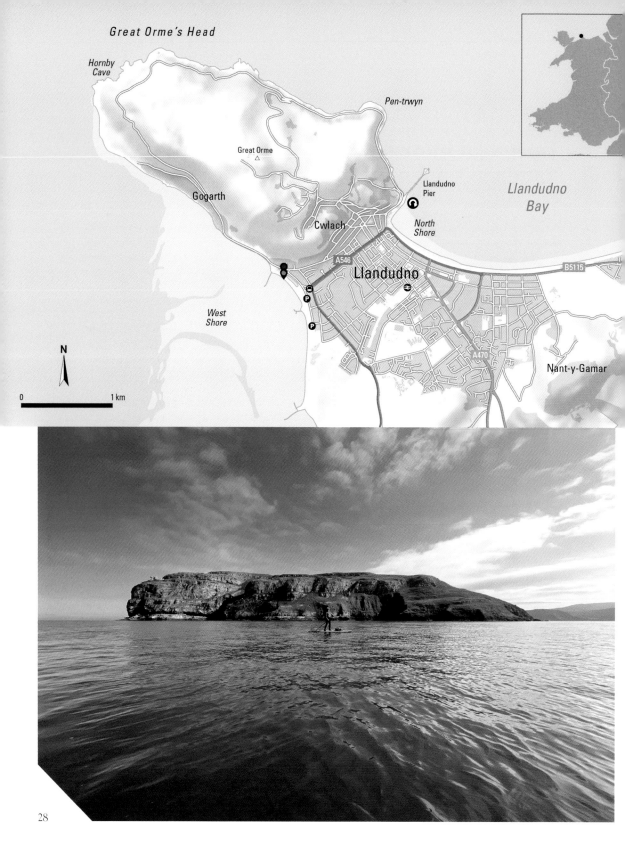

Great Orme's Head

Hornby
Cave

Pen-trwyn

Great Orme
△

Gogarth

Llandudno
Pier

*Llandudno
Bay*

Cwlach

North
Shore

A546

Llandudno

B5115

West
Shore

P

P

A470

Nant-y-Gamar

N

0   1 km

Llandudno West and North Shore, Great Orme

AN OLD GUIDEBOOK, CLAPOTIS, LLANDUDNO PIER AND PORPOISES IN THE GLISTENING SEA

'So when we reach the headland we may experience some *clapotis*,' says Caz, briefing me on our way to our coastal SUP adventure.

'Clafoutis?' I reply, somewhat perplexed as my mind wanders to memories of the delicious baked cherry cakes I'd tasted on my visits to France.

'No, *clapotis*. It's French for "lapping". It's where a wave hitting the vertical cliff comes back out and meets an incoming wave. When that happens, it looks like the waves are simply going up and down in the same spot, neither going in nor out. I read about it in an old canoeing guidebook, *Snowdonia White Water, Sea and Surf,* that I found in a second-hand bookshop. Cool, isn't it?' she explains enthusiastically.

I'm with Caz Dawson on our way to Llandudno's West Shore in North Wales to paddle round the famous Great Orme to the town's North Shore, using the ebb and flood of the tide to help us on our journey. I first met Caz, founder of SUP Lass Paddle Adventures, at the beginning of my research for this book, when she and her partner Jonathan shared the River Dee and Llyn Tegid with me (p23). I'm looking forward to catching up and hearing about her success in the Trent100 and her training for the upcoming Great Glen Challenge, an endurance race across Scotland.

Llandudno, often known as the queen of Welsh resorts, is a seaside town on the North Wales coastline in Conwy. Purpose-built in the late 1840s by the Mostyn family and the architect Owen Williams, it sits on the Creuddyn peninsula, looking out over the Irish Sea. There are two beaches, West Shore and North Shore. The former is the quieter of the two and lies on the estuary of the Afon Conwy. North Shore is a curving, three-kilometre-long beach flanked by the Great Orme on one side and the Little Orme on the other. With its Victorian promenade, lined by hotels and full of beautiful architecture, it has been a holiday destination for visitors to enjoy the sea air since the late 1800s. Alice Liddell and her family, believed to have been the inspiration for Lewis Carroll's *Alice's Adventures in Wonderland,* summered here. The Llandudno Pier, built in 1878, is a Grade-II-listed building and is the longest pier in Wales.

While just a kilometre and a half separates the two beaches by road along Gloddaeth Street or Gloddaeth Avenue, our plan is to paddle along the coastline from West Shore to North Shore and back, approximately 10 kilometres each way.

The Great Orme is a headland made up of limestone and dolomite, considered to be over 330 million years old. Some say its name comes from the Old Norse word for worm or sea serpent, *urm*. The cliffs rise over 207 metres above the sea, and the headland measures over three kilometres long and a kilometre and a half wide. Parts of the Great Orme are managed as a nature reserve, and it is also a Special Area of Conservation, Site of Special Scientific Interest and Heritage Coast.

Fulmars, kittiwakes, guillemots and razorbills nest here and on the way we see cormorants on the rock, drying their wings after diving for fish. Two species of butterfly have adapted to the

Opposite The Great Orme

fauna on the headland: the silver-studded blue and grayling butterflies appear earlier in the year than other species to feed on the grasses and flowers growing in the limestone. The Great Orme is also home to a herd of Kashmiri goats that have roamed the rugged cliffs for over a hundred years, recognisable by their huge, curved horns.

It is a slightly overcast morning as we launch from the beach and paddle towards the headland and area of *clapotis*. Paddleboarding gives us an excellent view of the caves along the cliffs of the Great Orme, including Hornby Cave, the site where the brig (a two-masted, square-rigged ship) *Hornby*, bound for South America from Liverpool, was shipwrecked on New Year's Day in 1824. High above us, we spot Llandudno's lighthouse, built in 1862 and now a guest house.

The colour of the water is striking and different to anything I have paddled on before: a turquoise green with a glistening, glass-like sheen despite the cloud. A couple of seals follow us, ducking and diving as we paddle along chatting. Using her coastal skills, Caz has timed our adventure to take advantage of the rising tide carrying us towards North Shore, and after two and a half hours of leisurely paddling we reach the north of the headland with the pier in our sights. Passengers on the Llandudno tourist boat, with its brightly coloured bunting, wave at us as they pass.

After a peek in Dutchman's Cave we head towards the majestic pier, picking up some litter from the sea along the way. Caz points out the Happy Valley Gardens where the Welsh National Eisteddfod ceremonies were held in 1896 and 1963. We can see people enjoying the

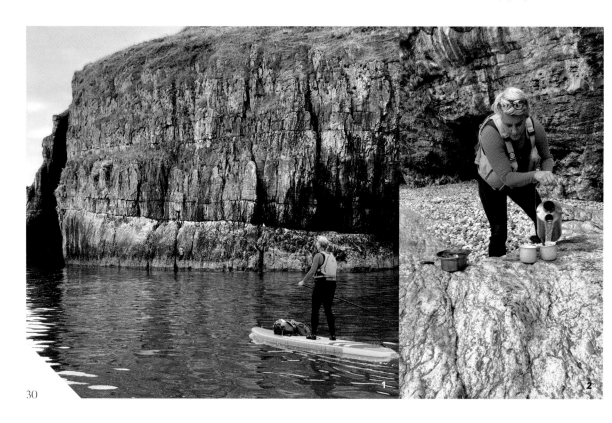

1 Caz paddling around the Great Orme   **2** Hot chocolate break   **3** Heading towards West Shore

gardens and the cable cars rising to the summit.

I had hoped to take a photo of Caz by the pier, but the tide has now turned and I can feel the pull of the water quite forcefully under my paddleboard. We are both looking forward to a little picnic and turn back to West Shore, stopping at a small beach to do a #2MinuteBeachClean of discarded remnants of barbecue parties that we pack away in our dry bags. After freshly made Kelly Kettle hot chocolate and biscuits we head back under blue skies. Shortly before reaching the headland we watch in wonder as two porpoises swim by.

In the distance, we can just see the outline of Anglesey and the Menai Strait. A couple of very experienced kayakers pass us, asking about the route we have taken – they know Caz from social media. I stand there beaming with pride at her planning and guiding skills as we talk through our Great Orme adventure.

After a cooling dip in the warm Irish Sea we are soon back at West Shore beach, now busy with families splashing in the waves and paddleboarders enjoying the shallow waters. There is a Mr Whippy van parked next to Caz's car, and a 99 ice cream with her name on it.

Driving past the beautiful hotels along the promenade on North Shore on our way home, I can see why Llandudno is so loved. It would be a dream to return, paddle around the pier again and explore the Little Orme. One for the wish list. You never know the adventures, learning or joy that will unfold from a canoeing guidebook found in a second-hand bookshop. I'm so grateful Caz was curious enough to buy it and share the Great Orme with me.

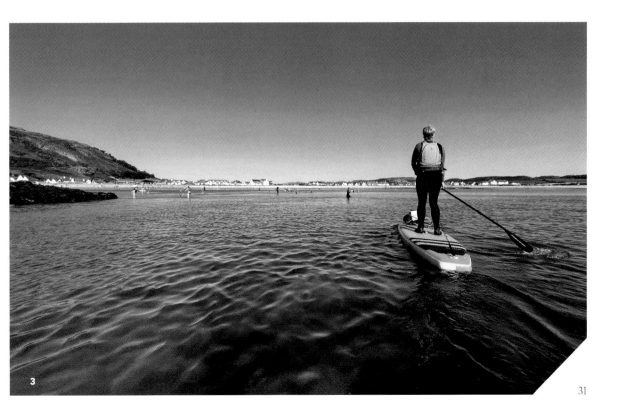

Technical information

DISTANCE **18.5km round trip.**

....

LAUNCH LOCATION:
ENTRY AND EXIT POINT **SH 770821/53.321, -3.847**
TURN AROUND POINT **SH 784828/53.328, -3.827**

Difficulty

I have included this trip as an example of what is possible when you have built up your skills, knowledge and experience – it is not one to take lightly. My recommendation would be to go on a guided tour with a qualified instructor who has experience of coastal planning – I felt safe under Caz's guidance, and she is trained and qualified as a VHF radio operator. There are courses available to build up your own coastal expedition skills and knowledge.

There are very few exit points along the cliff face around the Great Orme. If you have built up your technical skills and coastal knowledge, an option would be to paddleboard from one shore to the other as a one-way trip. Leave a car or catch a bus to the launch point. Paddleboarding close to the beaches would still be lovely and you would have the opportunity of two different beaches in one day.

Getting there

There are railway stations at Llandudno and Llandudno Junction. Buses to Bangor and Conwy can be caught just behind West Shore. Alternatively, National Express offers direct services to Llandudno from cities throughout the UK.

There is free parking on West Parade by West Shore (SH 773817/53.319, -3.843). There is also a car park on Dale Road (SH 773815/53.317, -3.843).

Route information

There is a webcam of West Shore at the West Shore Beach Cafe on Dale Road.

Eating and drinking

» West Shore Beach Cafe serves breakfast and lunch.
» The Lilly Restaurant on West Parade (there are public toilets just near here).

Instruction, guided tours and equipment hire

» SUP Lass Paddle Adventures, founded by Caz Dawson, offers beginner and improver classes, SUP socials, guided tours and coastal adventure planning.
» Psyched Paddleboarding, founded by Sian Sykes, offers beginner and improver classes, guided tours, coastal adventure planning, board hire and overnight camps in Anglesey and Snowdonia.

Further information

» Trent100 is a team challenge covering 100km in 20 hours across Staffordshire, Derbyshire and Nottinghamshire: *www.trent100.com*
» Terry Storry, *Snowdonia White Water, Sea and Surf: A canoeing guide* (Cicerone Press, 1987).
» The Great Glen Challenge is a challenge to paddleboard 92km of the Great Glen in either one or two days: *www.paddlefast. co.uk/greatglenchallenge*

Opposite Caz paddling around Llandudno **Overleaf** Sunset at Oxwich Bay © Shutterstock/Stephm2506

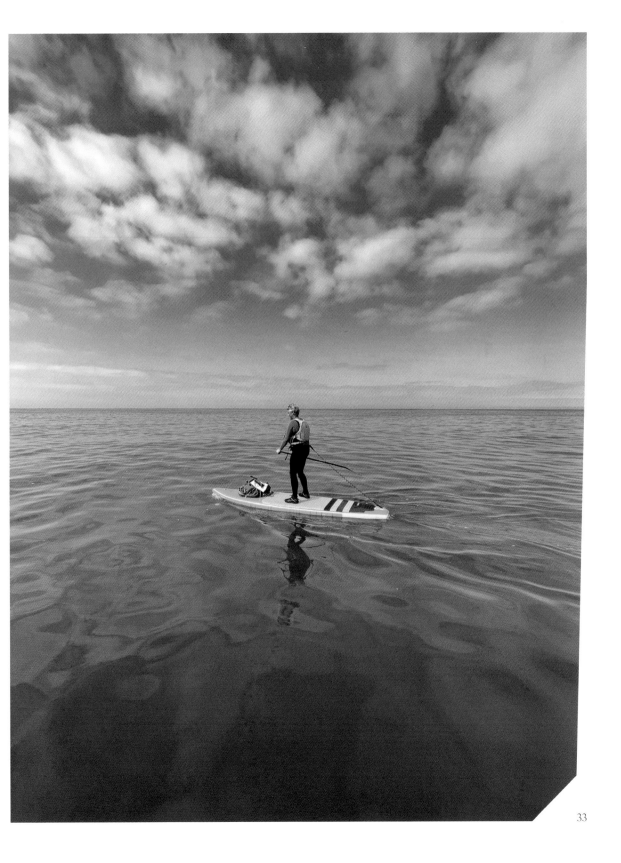

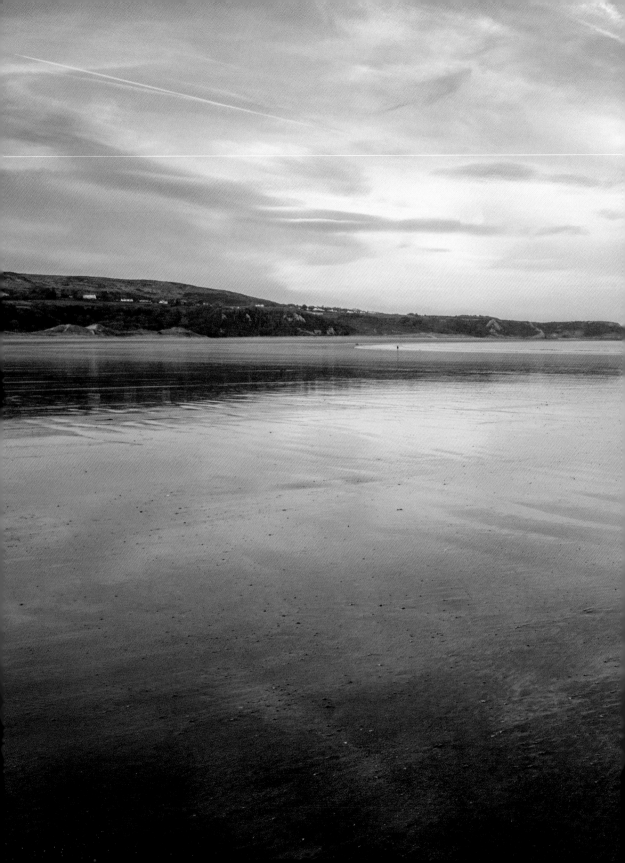

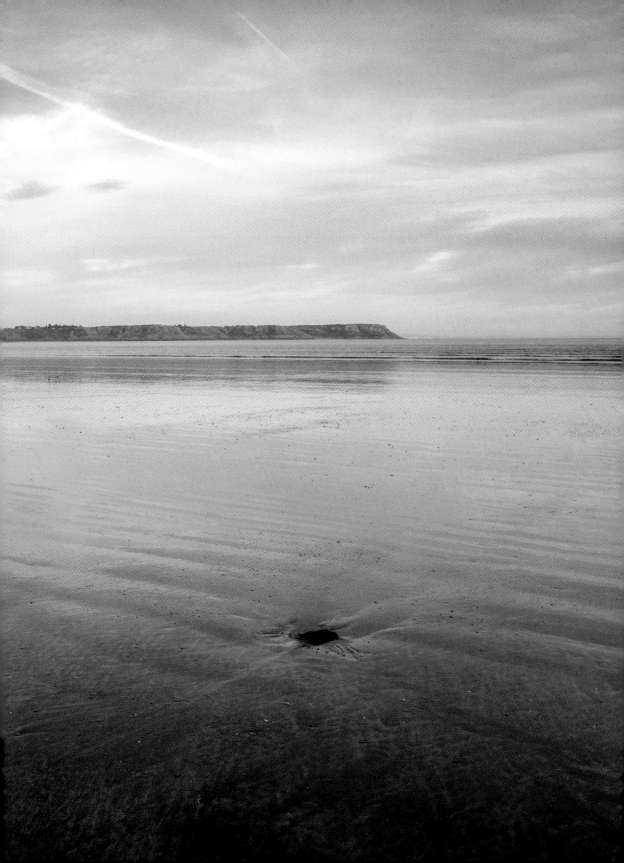

I remember arriving on the east coast at the start of my Scottish research and walking to the beach at Kingsbarns. The murmur of friends chatting by their tents reminded me that, due to the Land Reform (Scotland) Act 2003, responsible wild camping was allowed. What a treat to sleep under the stars.

I smile remembering the adventures I enjoyed: exploring the East Neuk of Fife (p71), a castle at St Andrews (p71) and then on to Loch Tay (p65). From there, I travelled north to Loch Morlich (p59), then on to mighty Loch Ness (p59).

Next up was Oban, where I paddled to Kerrera, my first solo SUP to an island (p47). I recall dancing round the kitchen as I booked a day on Mull (p53).

My final stop was Largs as I made my way home (p41). How incredibly lucky I was to be a part of this Scottish adventure.

All of this was still to come when I arrived in Kingsbarns, and an early night beckoned. The next morning, I left the village completely underestimating the magic that was about to unfold.

SCOTLAND

Opposite A sunset paddle to Great Cumbrae, Portencross and Largs, the Cumbraes
Overleaf Paddling just by St Andrews, St Andrews and the East Neuk of Fife © Paul Hutchison, @onthekillerwhaletrail

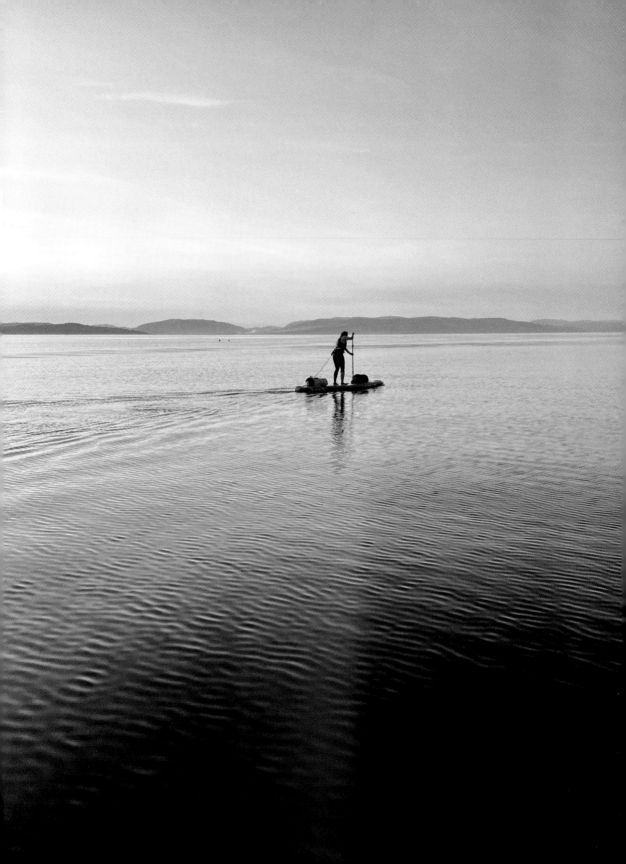

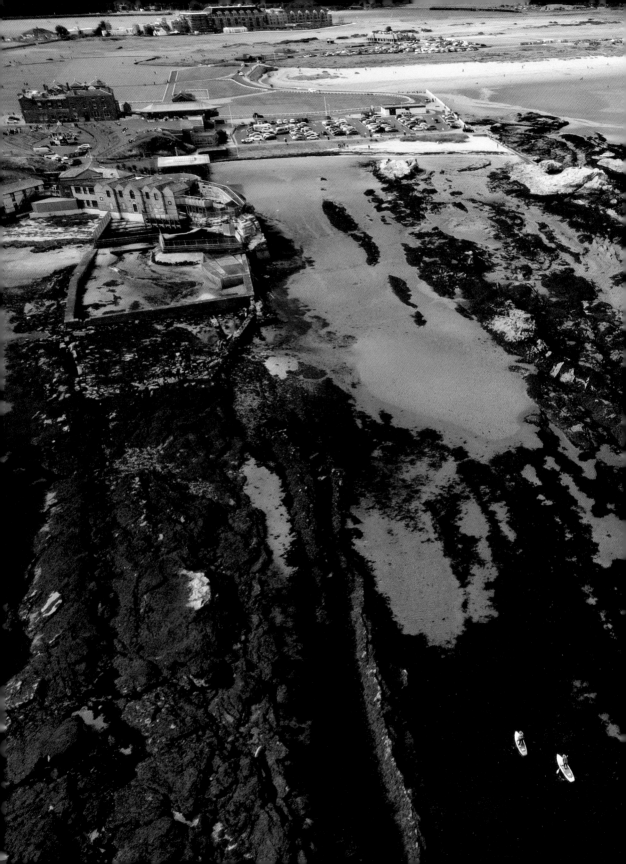

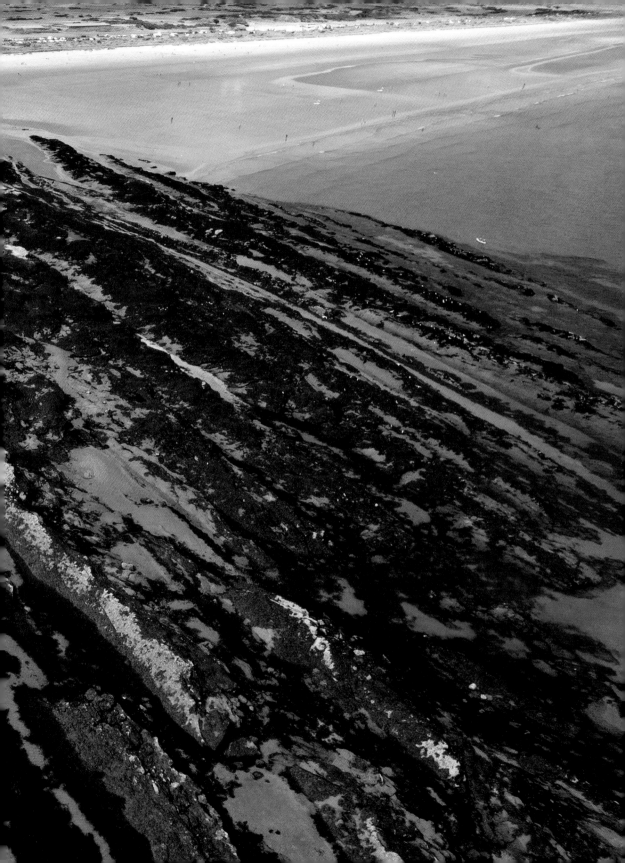

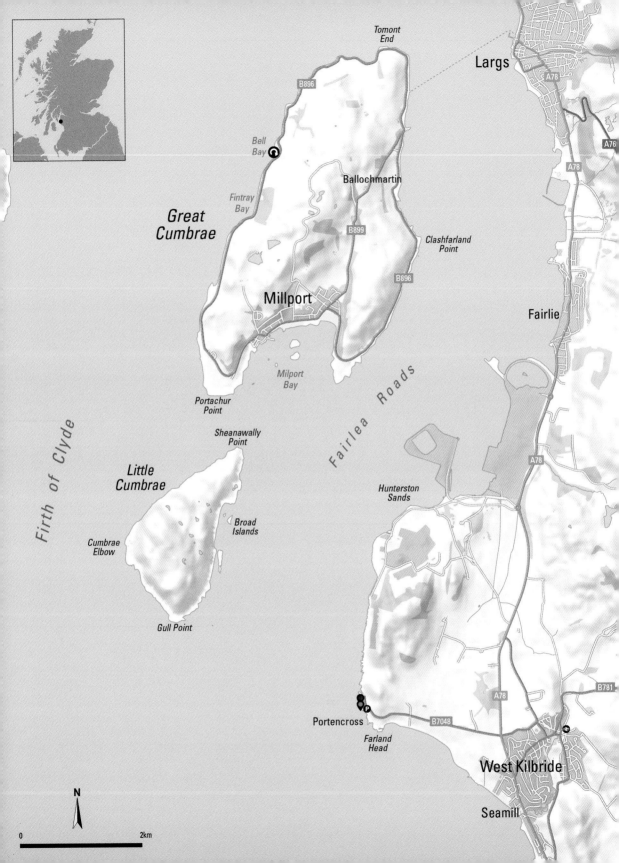

Tomont
End

Largs

B896

Bell
Bay

Ballochmartin

Fintray
Bay

Great
Cumbrae

B899

Clashfarland
Point

A78

A76

A78

B896

Fairlie

Millport

Milport
Bay

Portachur
Point

Fairlea Roads

Firth of Clyde

Sheanawally
Point

Little
Cumbrae

Hunterston
Sands

A78

Broad
Islands

Cumbrae
Elbow

Gull Point

B781

Portencross

B7048

A78

Farland
Head

West Kilbride

N

Seamill

0   2km

Portencross and Largs, the Cumbraes

SLEEPING ON A SUP, VIEWS TO ARRAN, STARFISH AND PASTA ON THE BEACH

'Hello, Jo! The weather for Sunday is looking dreadful, but it's beautiful the next day. Would you be up for a microadventure under the stars on Great Cumbrae as it will be a very warm night on Monday? Or we can stick to the original plan and push through the rain if need be?'

A message has just arrived from Linn van der Zanden, a SUP instructor based near Largs on the Firth of Clyde in north Ayrshire who works in education and also volunteers with young people. A rainy Sunday outing or sleeping on the beach on the west coast of Scotland on Monday? I wonder if you can guess my reply.

The afternoon sun sparkles on the sea as we meet at the car park near Portencross Castle, 14.5 kilometres south of Largs and five and a half kilometres west of West Kilbride. According to the castle's website, Portencross may have been the last resting place of the great kings of Scotland, as it was where they lay in state before being taken to Iona for burial.

With careful planning and Linn's excellent packing, we set off from the tiny inlet by the castle with our boards loaded for a SUP sleepout and head towards Little (or Wee) Cumbrae. Now privately owned, this is the smaller of the two islands known as the Cumbraes that lie between the Isle of Bute to the west, Arran to the south-west and the mainland to the east. It is a rocky island, formed from volcanic lava flow, with steep cliffs, and measures just under three kilometres long and a kilometre and a half wide. The Old Lighthouse, one of two on the island, was built in 1757 and is the second oldest lighthouse in Scotland. As we paddle past we can see the beautiful Little Cumbrae House, with gardens designed by Gertrude Jekyll, and then the old castle keep, standing on its own tidal islet.

The water is glassy and we take our time chatting, spotting jellyfish and birds as well as seals diving. We can just about see seals resting on their haul-out site on the shoreline and keep a good distance so we don't disturb them. Paddling side by side in the sunshine, Linn tells me how she started paddleboarding in 2017 when her daughter was three. After reading Alastair Humphreys's book *Microadventures*, she was inspired to start a project with friends to add more local, small adventures to her life around her busy career and family commitments. She swims, sails, has recently taken up surfing and enjoys SUP bivvy nights near her home in Ayrshire. She is also a Surfers Against Sewage representative, caring for the ocean that clearly brings her so much joy, and volunteers with the Ocean Youth Trust Scotland as well as supporting Cal Major's charity Seaful.

We pass the northerly tip of Little Cumbrae and paddle towards Great Cumbrae, where we can see Millport, the only town on the island. The island, which is six and a half kilometres long and three kilometres wide, is reached by ferry from nearby Largs. With sheltered bays, it is great for SUP and is also popular with cyclists enjoying the 16-kilometre circuit around the island.

As we paddle along the west coast, we look down through the crystal-clear waters and are amazed by the number of starfish (also known now as sea stars) and sea urchins below. While

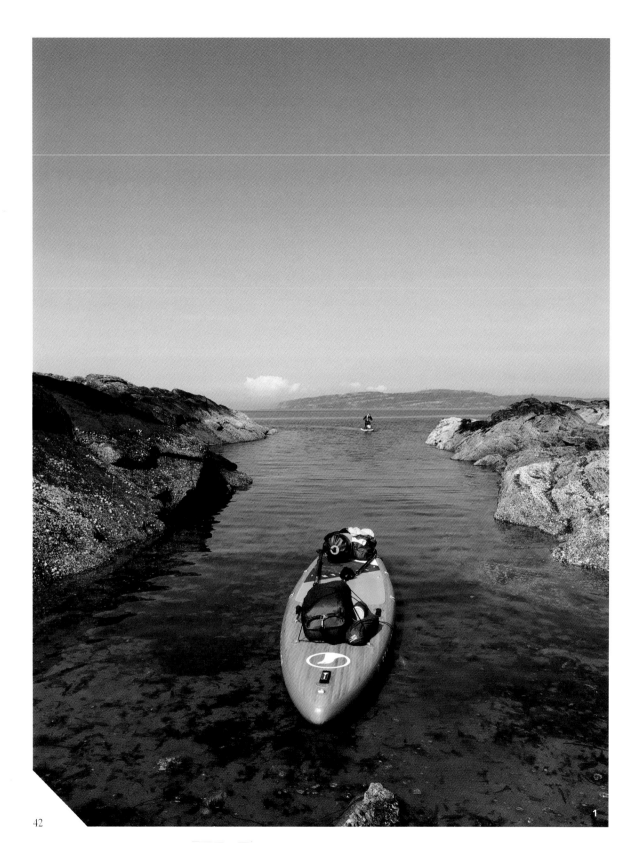

1

marvelling at the sea life here, Linn explains more about nearby Arran's Community Marine Reserve 'No Take Zone'. After campaigning by the Community of Arran Seabed Trust (COAST), an area of two and a half square kilometres of sea and seabed in the south Arran Marine Protected Area (MPA) in Lamlash Bay was established in 2008 as a 'No Take Zone'. The first of its kind in Scotland, this means no marine life can be taken from the area, including the shore, by commercial or recreational fishing. A post on COAST's website stated that research has revealed a 'dramatic increase (approx. 80%) in marine life abundance in the seas around Arran'.

The island's mountains are now a beautiful silhouette in the evening sun behind us and I keep turning round to soak up the stunning view, imagining what it would be like to paddle there.

One for the wish list. A few minutes later a boat passes in the distance and we spot dolphins ahead. We stand and watch in quiet awe as they swim by.

It's time to set up camp for the night, and we choose Bell Bay Beach, making sure we carry our boards above the tide line – high tide is at 2 a.m. and we don't want to take any chances. I'm so grateful that Linn really has brought everything: we each have an inflatable mattress on top of our boards, bivvy bag and sleeping bag. She kindly gives me a mosquito tent which I slide through the D rings on my board, while she will use a head net to keep the midges away.

Supper is soon on the go – pasta, pesto and pine nuts – which we warm on the Kelly Kettle, followed by a soothing mug of peppermint tea and dark chocolate. It's difficult to describe

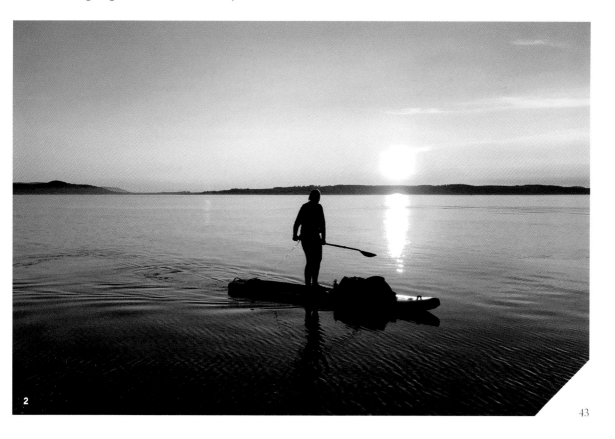

quite how perfect it feels, sharing stories, watching the light fade and hearing the waves lapping on the shore in the darkness. After 11 kilometres of paddling, I snuggle into my eldest son's sleeping bag on my board Grace, wearing my youngest son's padded jacket for extra warmth, and am quickly asleep. A couple of hours later I wake up, startled, thinking I'm at home and someone has switched the light on. After a few moments, I remember I'm on a beach in Scotland and the bright light is in fact the moon. I say a little thank you for the experience and drift back off into my dreams.

After the sunshine of the day before, we wake to a misty morning. I had confidently told Linn I would be up at my usual 6.30 a.m. but actually sleep in until 7.40 a.m. as my makeshift bed was so comfy, something I had not expected. Breakfast is soaked oats and dried fruit and then we pack up camp. We both want to make sure we leave no trace and do a #2MinuteBeachClean, leaving this special spot

cleaner than we found it. We can hear a foghorn in the distance and paddle back to Portencross along the same route we came, as the sun burns through the cloud.

Two and half hours later, our boards are packed away and we are ready to return to our work and families, with sand in our hair, our hearts full and a new friendship formed. On my way home I text Alastair Humphreys to tell him about Linn, the joy his book has brought her and the evening we shared on our own beach microadventure.

'That's so cool!' he replies. I smile – it has indeed been very cool.

A guiding principle when researching this book has been to share the possibilities of paddleboarding – the stories of place, people and SUP experiences. I had not envisaged that one day it would include sleeping overnight on a Scottish island. A night under the stars I shall never forget.

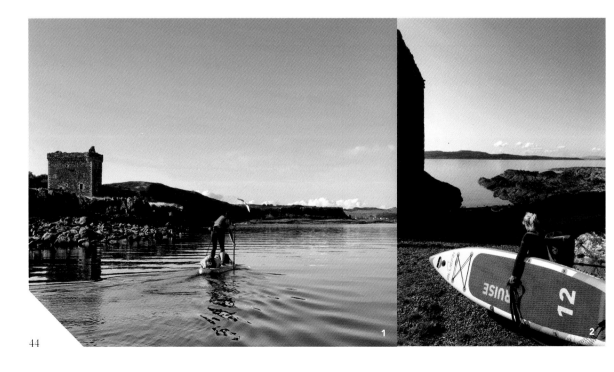

1 Paddling around Little Cumbrae   2 Setting off from Portencross Castle © @microadventuregirl
3 Our camp for the night on Great Cumbrae

Technical information

DISTANCE **22.6km round trip.**

LAUNCH LOCATION
ENTRY AND EXIT POINT **NS 176489/55.699, -4.905**
TURN AROUND POINT **NS 163577/55.777, -4.931**

ALTERNATIVE ROUTES **A shorter route of 1.5km each way would be launching from the Largs Yacht Haven car park to Ballochmartin Bay, or from Portencross to the south tip of Little Cumbrae.**
   A route of 5km each way would be launching from Aubrey Pond, north of Largs, to Fintray Bay on Great Cumbrae.
   Paddleboarding on Great Cumbrae, at Portencross Beach and nearby Seamill beach would be a lovely alternative.

Difficulty
Paddleboarding experience is necessary for this trip and knowledge of wind and tides is important for the journey from Portencross to Great Cumbrae.

Getting there
West Kilbride can be reached by frequent buses from Largs, Ayr and Ardrossan, and has a railway station with direct connections to Glasgow and Largs. Frequent buses to Ayr also stop on the A78. From here it is just under 3km to the launch point.
   There is a car park at Portencross just by the castle (NS 177488/55.698, -4.903) which is 300m from the launch point.

Eating and drinking
» On Great Cumbrae, the seasonal Fintry Bay Cafe is close to Bell Bay Beach.
» The Waterside Hotel on Ardrossan Road, West Kilbride is not far from Portencross Castle.

Instruction, guided tours and equipment hire
» Ayrshire Paddle Sports, based in Ardrossan, offers paddleboarding lessons, tours and social SUP sessions in north Ayrshire. It will be running tours to Great Cumbrae.
» Glasgow Paddleboarders Co is a team of freelance instructors offering guided tours, lessons and paddleboard sales.
» You can hire kayaks from On Your Bike Millport on Great Cumbrae.

Further information
» Community of Arran Seabed Trust (COAST): *www.arrancoast.com*
» Seaful: *www.seaful.org.uk*
» Surfers Against Sewage: *www.sas.org.uk*
» Alastair Humphreys, *Microadventures: Local discoveries for great escapes* (William Collins, 2014).
» Kula Cloth, antimicrobial pee cloths (*www.kulacloth.com*), are available in the UK from SUP endurance adventurer Shells Ellison: *www.shellsellison.com*
» Ocean Youth Trust Scotland: *www.oytscotland.org.uk*

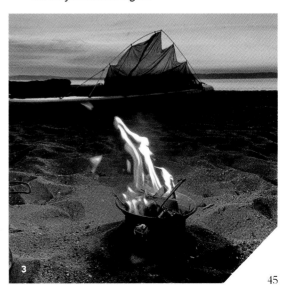

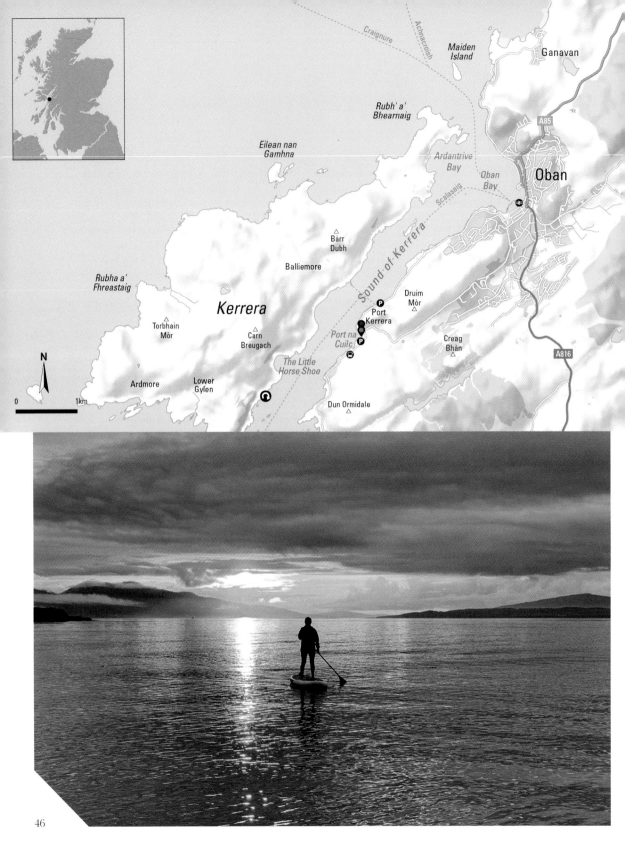

Sound of Kerrera and Ganavan Sands, Oban

A HEBRIDEAN ISLAND ADVENTURE, GOLDEN SEAWEED AND PINK URCHINS, SEALS AND SUNDAY BREAKFAST BY THE BEACH

The late-afternoon sun sparkles on the water as I float along the edge of Sound of Kerrera, watching the golden seaweed swaying gently beneath. Checking it is safe to do so, I lie on my back, close my eyes and exhale. The soothing 'tut, tut' of my board on the sea is all I can hear as I bathe in the sunlight.

'Thank you,' I whisper, 'thank you for this moment.' Nobody will hear my thanks, except perhaps my soul. It is a tiny ritual I practise every time I paddleboard, wherever I am and whomever I'm with. A way to capture the joy for those days when the world seems at its harshest and the days the most difficult. I treasure today for those tomorrows.

'That looks like a heavenly spot to camp,' I say to a couple pottering around their red tent on the grass above a few minutes later.

'It is,' they reply, smiling. 'It's perfect. Just perfect.'

I am just under five kilometres south of Oban, the 'gateway to the Isles' in the Scottish Highlands region of Argyll and Bute, just past the Puffin Dive Centre at Gallanach where I launched three hours earlier. I have come to Oban to paddle to the island of Kerrera, as recommended by paddleboarder and author Matt Gambles, to explore Ganavan Sands north of the town and take a day trip to Mull on the CalMac ferry (p53).

Oban is a bustling seaside town in a horseshoe-shaped bay, surrounded by forests, gardens and mountains. The Dunollie and Dunstaffnage castles rest nearby and Castle

Stalker is further north. There is also a whisky distillery, museums and galleries. Five and a half kilometres out of town lies the Ocean Explorer Centre, the visitor centre to the Scottish Association for Marine Science, which is Scotland's oldest independent marine science organisation.

Protecting Oban Bay from the Atlantic Ocean is the island of Kerrera, approximately six and a half kilometres long and three kilometres wide. Only vehicles owned by the residents (68 full-time residents including 19 children as of June 2019) are allowed on the island, making it a perfect place for walkers to enjoy the stunning Hebridean scenery.

You can travel the 600 metres from the mainland to Kerrera by MV *Carvoria*, CalMac's smallest ferry which carries just 12 people. Alternatively, as I am about to do, you can paddleboard across.

For a small fee, the Puffin Dive Centre offers parking and use of its toilets, showers and hot drinks as well as easy access from the slipway. It also looks after the #2MinuteBeachClean station we worked together to fund after my coast-to-coast challenge.

I feel quite the adventurer as I push off from the slipway into the clear, warm waters of the Firth of Lorn for my first 'mainland to island' SUP trip. Around 15 minutes later, I reach the coastline of Kerrera and paddle southwards in the sunshine, stopping off at Horse Shoe and then Little Horse Shoe Bay. An old shipwreck lies on its side, the rust-coloured timbers and golden seaweed adding a rich contrast to the blue of the sky. Trees grow close to the pebbly shore and sheep graze on the hill above. I start

Opposite Beautiful light at Ganavan Sands

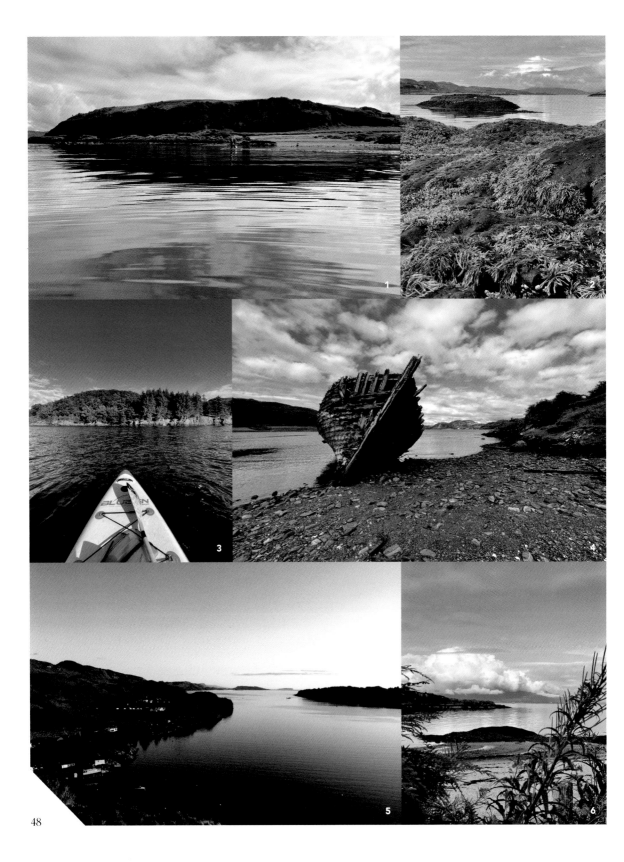

48

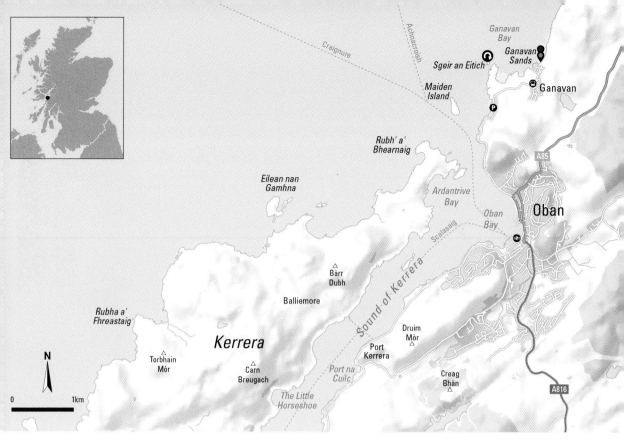

imagining a week here, exploring the different beaches from the sea, reading, writing and eating picnics.

On the south coast of Kerrera lies Gylen Castle, the castle of fountains, built in 1582. With its oriel window and vaulted cellar, this would be a great adventure for another day with more time, planning and snacks. As I bob along, sitting on my board and dangling my feet in the water, I am aware of three curious seals diving and popping up nearby. I keep my distance, turn and paddle across to the other side of the sound on my way back to the centre, passing the happy couple in the tent on the way, in awe of the beauty beneath the water. Three hours of simple, soulful, slow paddling before returning to thank my friends at Puffin Dive Centre.

Later that evening I walk along the harbour front and by chance join a group of people quietly enthralled by an otter playing on the rocks. It's the end to a truly glorious late summer's day.

After a blustery day on Mull (p53) and a day resting and writing, I'm about to visit my second destination here, Ganavan Sands, four kilometres north of Oban. It has been raining for 36 hours, but with little wind and a tiny sliver of blue sky I remain hopeful. I park right by the beach and start pumping my board, listening to the sound of sizzling sausages being fried in front of the campervan nearby. Children are building sandcastles and a family swim together in the sea.

Three couples, one with two children, launch from the beach at the same time as me, one heading for Dunstaffnage Castle, another round the corner to Little Ganavan. It's now bright blue skies and sunshine. The clarity of

1 Paddling out from Ganavan Sands 2 Seaweed at Ganavan Sands
3 Looking towards the mainland, with Kerrera behind 4 The shipwreck at Little Horse Shoe Bay
5 Looking across the Sound of Kerrera © Imogen Broad, Puffin Dive Centre 6 Ganavan Sands

1 A break on Kerrera

the light and views from my board across to Lismore, Morven and Mull are breathtaking – to think yesterday it had been shrouded in grey and rain. I paddle along the shore, watching hikers along the coastal path. A beautiful, pink sea urchin catches my eye and for a few minutes I admire it as the waves gently lap the rocks. Sometimes we paddle hard, sometimes we simply pootle along.

Heading back to the beach I meet the couple that I had been pumping my board by. We sit and chat on the sea in the sunshine as they tell me of the adventures SUP has opened up for them to learn, explore and enjoy together. This is just the beginning of their paddleboarding journey and I am as excited for them as I am for my own.

I return to the beach and deflate my board, amazed at the blue skies after so much rain. The bay is fuller now with hikers, sandcastle builders, dippers and sunbathers enjoying a Sunday afternoon by the sea.

It is time to say goodbye to Oban and head south to Largs, stopping to admire Loch Lomond on the way. I am grateful to have experienced just a tiny bit of what this coastline and the Inner Hebrides offer paddleboarders. I will definitely be back to explore and do hope you will be too.

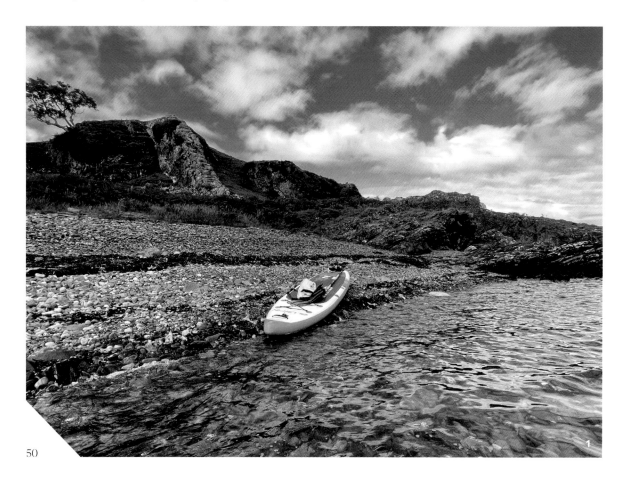

1

Technical information

DISTANCE
SOUND OF KERRERA **6km round trip.**
GANAVAN SANDS **5km round trip.**

LAUNCH LOCATION
SOUND OF KERRERA
ENTRY AND EXIT POINT **NM 832277/56.392, -5.514**
TURN AROUND POINT **NM 817268/56.383, -5.539**
GANAVAN SANDS
ENTRY AND EXIT POINT **NM 862327/56.438, -5.469**
TURN AROUND POINT **NM 853328/56.438, -5.484**

ALTERNATIVE ROUTES **Paddleboarding close to the Puffin Dive Centre would be a beautiful paddle. You could take the ferry to Kerrera and paddle back. Also, keeping close to Ganavan Sands would be a lovely trip.**

Difficulty
An understanding of tides and wind is important for paddleboarding on the sea.

Getting there
Sound of Kerrera
There is a railway station in Oban, with direct trains to Glasgow. Megabus and Citylink routes run from Glasgow to Oban. There is also a bus from Oban to the Oban Camping and Caravanning Park, 300m from the launch point.

For a small fee you can park at Puffin Dive Centre (NM 831277/56.392, -5.514) and use its showers and toilets as well as make hot drinks. The slipway offers an easy launch point. Alternatively, there is some parking by Kerrera ferry port (NM 835283/56.397, -5.510).

Ganavan Sands
From Oban it is just under 4km along from the Corran Esplanade. A bus from Oban runs regularly to Ganavan.

There is a pay-and-display car park at Ganavan Sands (NM 862327/56.438, -5.469). This is right by the beach and makes launching straightforward. There are public toilets nearby.

Eating and drinking
» I had a delicious breakfast at the Little Potting Shed Cafe on John Street in Oban and bought things for my picnic from Go Naked Veg on Stevenson Street.
» Dougie Dan's burger van in the Ganavan Sands car park serves meat and vegetarian burgers, snacks and hot drinks.

Instruction, guided tours and equipment hire
» You can hire boards, take lessons and have guided tours along the bays and coastline at the Puffin Dive Centre.
» Basking Shark Scotland offers tuition and guided tours from Oban and Mull.
» There are no facilities to hire boards or have lessons at Ganavan Sands. The closest is the Puffin Dive Centre.

Further information
» Kerrera: *www.isleofkerrera.org*
» Kerrera Tea Gardens and Bunkhouse: *www.kerrerabunkhouse.co.uk*

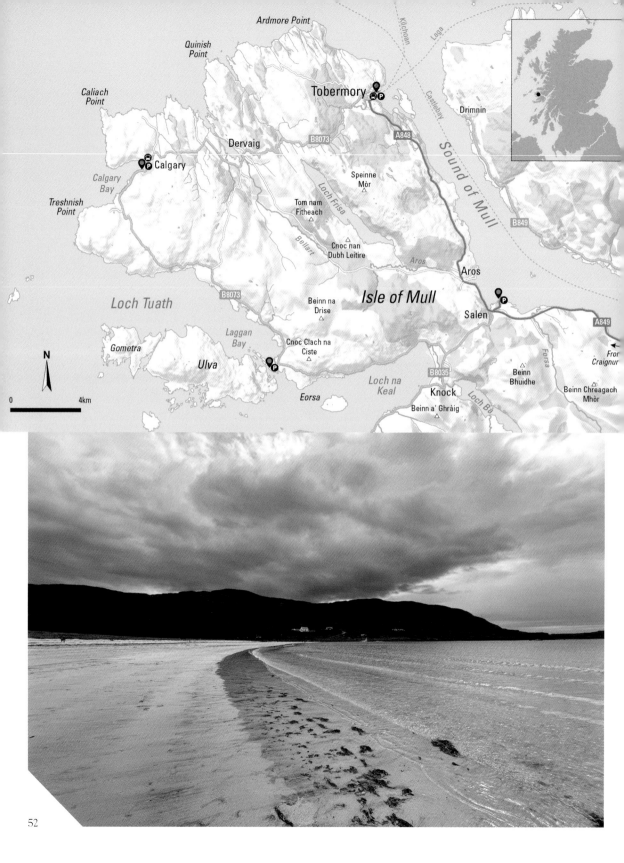

Isle of Mull

**WHITE, SANDY BEACHES, AN ISLAND FERRY,
PAINTED HOUSES AND WRITING BY THE FIRE**

My finger hovers over the button on the CalMac ferry booking site. A change to my plans means I have an unexpected extra day in Oban. There are spaces on the ferry to Mull if I set off early and return on the last sailing. Should I? Shouldn't I? I close my eyes, press 'make payment' and then do a little kitchen dance. I'm going to Mull, the second-largest island, after Skye, of the Inner Hebrides off the west coast of Scotland.

After a beautiful, sunny day on Sound of Kerrera (p47), exploring Oban and watching an otter at sunset, the next morning I board the ferry from Oban for the 46-minute journey to Craignure on Mull. Mull is approximately 38 kilometres from north to south and 41 kilometres west to east, with a coastline, including all its tiny bays, of over 482 kilometres. There are six castles and one Munro (a Scottish mountain over 3,000 feet) called Ben More. As a friend who visits regularly once told me, you can experience all the weathers in one day on Mull. The forecast is wind and rain for the next three days, so the chances of paddleboarding along the white sands and turquoise waters of Calgary Bay that I've been dreaming of since booking my ticket are small, but I remain hopeful.

Leaving the ferry, I enjoy a delicious breakfast at The Little Bespoke Bakery in Salen, then drive 16 kilometres north to the capital, Tobermory, and park near the harbour. I'd spent a lovely day here with my sons a few years ago and was excited to see the rainbow-coloured shops and homes again, which some of you may recall from CBeebies's *Balamory*. A lovely chap on social media, Nick Ray, a kayaker who lives on Mull, has kindly told me where to launch. I am good to go.

As I peer out of the car window, I soon realise that wherever I am going, it is not going to be on a paddleboard. Boats are swaying side to side on their moorings and the dark, grey sea is looking a tad choppy under ominous clouds.

Even if I can't paddleboard I can explore, and I set about finding four paddleboarding places to share with you. First a wander through Tobermory, visiting the Hebridean Whale and Dolphin Trust to learn about its work to protect the pilot whales, orcas, minke whales, dolphins and porpoises that swim in the Hebridean waters. Then it's the Mull Museum and finally I pop to the wonderful Tackle & Books bookshop for some postcards and a book on the Scottish coast. A few minutes later I'm up the hill at the An Tobar gallery and cafe where Eugenie, who works at the gallery, admires my Wave Project 'Surf Therapy' sweatshirt. When I tell her I'm here to paddleboard she says there is a new paddleboarding company in Tobermory and kindly sends me the details of Laura at Tobermory Paddle Hire.

It's time to head to Calgary Bay, around 20 kilometres west of Tobermory, with a quick stop for a cup of tea at The Piece Box at Dervaig, which sells homemade sandwiches, cakes and Isle of Mull ice cream. Calgary Bay is everything I dreamed of: a beautiful, sweeping stretch of white sands, low hills and trees as well as a scattering of pretty, white houses. The water is clear, chilly and utterly mesmerising. I watch a paddleboarder I met on the ferry go out on his board for about 10 minutes, get blown about and wisely return. Grace, my paddleboard, is definitely staying in the car today. At the back of the beach, there is a machair conservation area, designated a Site of Special Scientific Interest, to protect the fragile sand dunes and

Opposite The beach at Calgary Bay

coastal grassland called machair, a unique and rare habitat that is found on the exposed west-facing coastlines of Scotland and the Republic of Ireland. Red clover, bird's-foot-trefoil, yarrow and daisies grow within the machair in the calcium-rich sand.

Nearby is the seasonal Robin's Boat, selling snacks and Isle of Mull ice cream, where there is an information board about otters; it asks you to donate to children's education in Nepal in return for parking in the field.

I follow the road south, visiting the Cafe@CalgaryArts and art centre, where local artists' work is exhibited, and there is a sculpture trail through the woods and beach.

The views of the incoming weather in the distance are dramatic. I pause to listen to a waterfall and pass the famous Highland cattle,

with their shaggy coat and wide horns, grazing by the roadside.

My next stop is at the slipway for the Ulva ferry, and as I'm looking at the clear water and the tiny islands just off the shoreline, the ferry, driven by Rhuri Munro, arrives. His passenger for the short journey to Ulva is Brendan, who with his partner Mark runs The Boathouse Cafe on the island. With Mull's famous cheese platter on the menu and the beauty of Ulva, a community-owned island, this looks like a perfect place to paddle on a calm day.

I make my way south, stopping every so often to soak in the view, and meet a couple of very keen ornithologists who lend me their binoculars so I can see the white-tailed eagles they've been patiently watching. In 2020 there were 20 pairs on Mull, attracting many bird

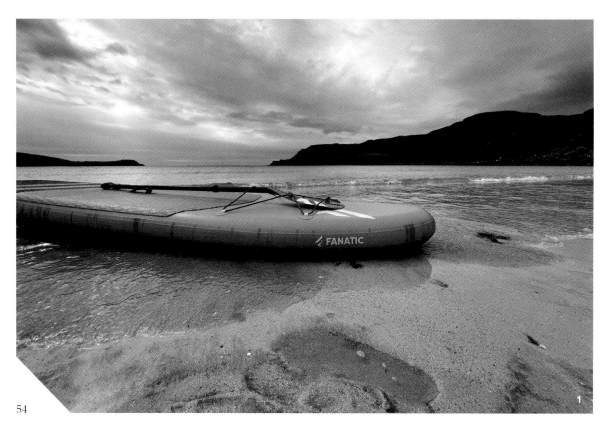

1

1 Calgary Bay   **2** The stunning beach at Calgary Bay   **3** Highland cow
4 Tobermory   **5** Boats floating near the Ulva ferry port

enthusiasts to the island. I don't quite realise how special it is to see them until the next day, so their generosity is very touching.

A few minutes later, I spot a board on the roof of a car as I pass a campsite and dash over to the owners, from Devon, to ask if they've had chance to paddleboard on Mull.

'Yesterday, in the sunshine,' they reply. 'The water was so clear, we almost felt dizzy we could see so far down.' Ah, heavenly.

I have one final destination to squeeze in – the Salen Bay Campsite, as I've heard it offers paddleboard hire. I meet Fergus and he tells me what a lovely bay it is to explore, as well as their plans for the future.

With my notebook full of ideas, I decide to call it a day as the evening is drawing in. The nearby Isle of Mull Hotel & Spa looks

inviting, and I'm grateful that for once I'm not in my neoprene leggings and rash vest. After a warm welcome, I'm soon sitting by the roaring fire with a nice cup of tea, reflecting upon the day.

Do I wish I had been able to paddleboard? Yes, I would love to share how my paddle was with you. Do I think I did the right thing by not paddleboarding? Also, yes: it was too windy to be safe. One of the things I admire most about endurance SUP adventurers such as Brendon Prince, Charlie Head, Cal Major, Sophie Witter and Dave Chant of SUP It and Sea, who all completed extraordinary challenges in 2021, is the emphasis on safety on the water as the priority. Knowing when to say 'if in doubt, don't go out,' as Simon from *SUPfm* podcast always mentions is part and parcel of our sport.

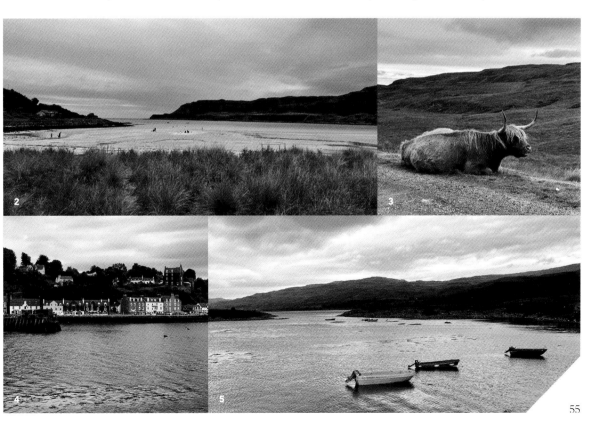

This has nevertheless been a magical day of beautiful views, dramatic weather and lovely conversations. I hope one day you and I will experience the dizzying joy of paddleboarding on Mull. As the fire crackles, I start writing my postcards from Tackle & Books. Wish you were here? Absolutely!

Technical information

```
DISTANCE
TOBERMORY HARBOUR 3km round trip.
ULVA 3km round trip.
CALGARY BAY 3km round trip.
SALEN 3km round trip.
......................................................................
LAUNCH LOCATION
TOBERMORY HARBOUR
ENTRY POINT NM 506553/56.623, -6.067
ULVA
ENTRY POINT NM 446399/56.482, -6.150
CALGARY BAY
ENTRY POINT NM 373509/56.577, -6.279
SALEN
ENTRY POINT NM 577438/56.524, -5.941
```

Difficulty
Although I did not paddle here, I think that with an understanding of tides and wind as well as good launch points these would be fairly interesting routes. Be sure to keep good distance from moored boats and the Ulva ferry, and keep in mind that conditions can change quickly.

Getting there
CalMac run ferries from Oban to Craignure, with tickets either with a vehicle or as a day passenger. There are sailings from Lochaline on Morvern and Kilchoan on the Ardnamurchan peninsula. When you reach the island, West Coast Motors bus services run throughout Mull.

Tobermory
The Tobermory Harbour car park is a pay and display (NM 504550/56.620, -6.069). Buses to Calgary and Craignure also stop here. There are public toilets, showers and washing machines available.

Ulva ferry port
There are two car parks – one is used primarily for the Ulva ferry (NM 446399/56.482, -6.147), so please use the car park just east of the ferry port (NM 447400/56.482, -6.147).

Calgary Bay
Free parking is available behind the beach (NM 374513/56.580, -6.278), and buses from Tobermory also stop a few times a day. There are public toilets nearby.

Salen
There is parking on the Salen Bay Campsite (NM 578437/56.523, -5.940), which runs paddleboard hire. The campsite offers self-launch opportunities, with a launch fee, alongside use of the showers/toilets.

Eating and drinking
 » An Tobar art gallery and cafe.
 » Robin's Boat serves drinks and ice cream.
 » The Piece Box in Dervaig offers sandwiches, drinks and homemade cakes.
 » Cafe@CalgaryArts.
 » The Boathouse.
 » The Little Bespoke Bakery serves breakfasts and lunches, pies, cakes and bread.
 » The Coffee Pot serves lunches, home baking and drinks.
 » The Isle of Mull Hotel & Spa is just under 1km from the ferry terminal at Craignure.

1 Looking out from the north-west coast of Mull towards Ulva

Instruction, guided tours and equipment

» You will need to bring your own board or hire from Tobermory.

» Laura Hewitt offers mobile paddleboard hire from Tobermory Beach.

» Basking Shark Scotland offers SUP tuition and guided tours from Oban and Mull.

» The owners of the Salen Bay Campsite offer paddleboard hire in conjunction with Salen Bay Hire.

Further information

» Ulva island community: *www.ulva.scot*

» Hebridean Whale and Dolphin Trust: *www.hwdt.org*

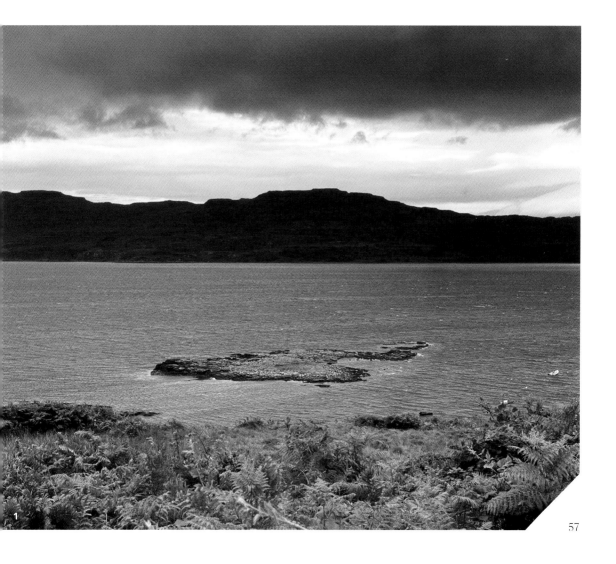

1

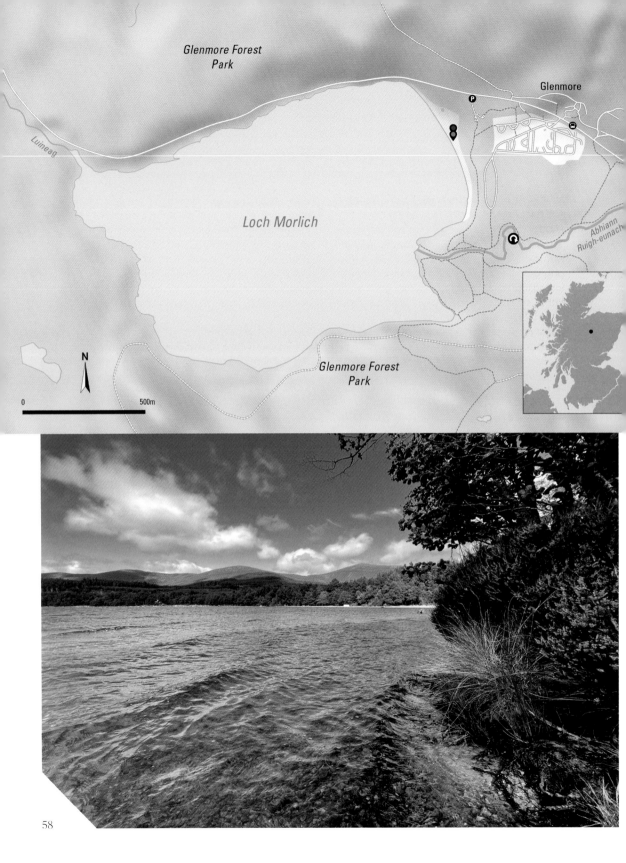

Loch Morlich and Loch Ness

BEACH LIFE IN THE MOUNTAINS, SOLO EXPLORING, THE GREAT GLEN CANOE TRAIL AND THE JOY OF PADDLING TOGETHER

'No, Daddy, just sit there!' she says, paddling with great determination into the wind. In her bright-orange buoyancy aid, her younger sister is working equally hard at the back while their father, smiling, shrugs his shoulders and replies, 'OK.' I've passed them before on the loch, admiring the tenacity of two little girls, perhaps eight and six years old, navigating the waters in their green Canadian canoe.

'Wow, you're doing brilliantly taking your dad on an adventure,' I say.

'I know!' replies the older girl proudly, momentarily looking up from her endeavours.

'How lucky am I?' adds their dad with a grin. They are making little progress on the waves, but they are undoubtedly making some very special memories together.

I'm on Loch Morlich, a freshwater loch at the foot of the northern Cairngorms in the Scottish Highlands, 204 kilometres north of Edinburgh and 10 kilometres from the popular ski-resort town of Aviemore. Surrounded by the Caledonian pines of Glenmore Forest Park and overlooked by Cairn Gorm and Ben Macdui, Loch Morlich's beach is advertised as the highest in Britain. Over 300 metres above sea level, it was the first beach on a freshwater loch to be awarded a Seaside Award by Keep Scotland Beautiful in 2009.

At 4,528 square kilometres, the Cairngorms is the largest national park in the UK, twice the size of the Lake District, and is home to four of the five highest mountains in Britain. Glenmore Forest Park is one of nine National Nature Reserves within the Cairngorms, and it is a beautiful spot to park and pump up my

board before a short walk through trees to the beach. It's a Tuesday afternoon in the middle of August and there are dippers in the shallow waves, ramblers, families on paddleboards and in canoes, people having picnics on the beach, swimmers with floats, snoozers in the sunshine and couples quietly engrossed in their books on deckchairs. The Boathouse Cafe and SUP hire are busy with customers and there are ice creams aplenty.

I launch into the breeze and make my way to the quieter end of the beach, just under a kilometre in the distance. The upturned roots of a tree, worn by the elements, mark the corner to a small river that feeds the loch called Abhainn Ruigh-eunachan, which I decide to explore. Twisting and turning through the woods, it widens and narrows, becomes shallow and then deepens. I paddle under a bridge, wishing a cheery hello to a couple hiking, and then follow the edge of an island. The water is a clear amber and warm to the skin as I wade through to pick up a discarded hard hat from the pebbled riverbed. Missing my footing, I stumble and am soon waist-deep, giggling to myself. Branches block the way here and there and I clamber over, pulling my board and enjoying the sense of freedom. A few minutes later I come across a family trying in vain to turn their canoe, laughing uncontrollably and apologising for holding me up. 'What happens on the water stays on the water,' I reassure them.

I return to the beach, passing the girls and their dad in the canoe, and enjoy a nice cup of tea among the pine trees, imagining a winter paddle on the loch with snow on the mountains above. Today has been a gentle, soul-nourishing, solo exploration along the beautiful Abhainn Ruigh-eunachan. A tiny adventure, yet huge joy.

Opposite Loch Morlich

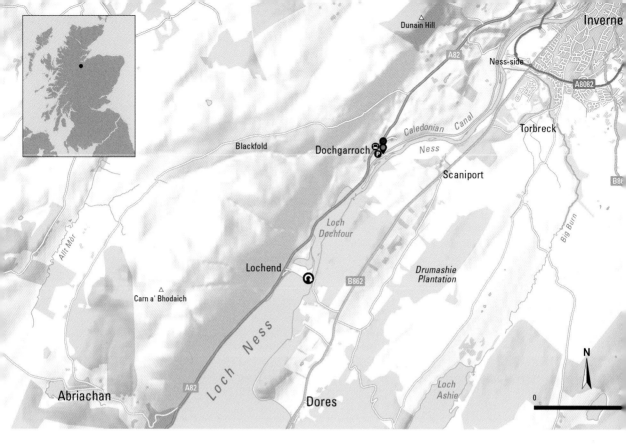

Tomorrow the Caledonian Canal and the mighty Loch Ness. Smiling as I recall the little girl's determination, I leave Loch Morlich and head north to Inverness.

From the start of my research, I knew I wanted to tell you about the Great Glen Canoe Trail, the magnificent, 96-kilometre, coast-to-coast journey from Fort William to Inverness which attracts approximately 4,000 canoeists, kayakers and paddleboarders a year. With Loch Lochy, Loch Oich, Loch Ness and Loch Dochfour as well as 35 kilometres of the man-made Caledonian Canal, choosing just one section amid the splendour was proving tricky. I messaged Fiona Quinn – who in 2018 became the first woman to complete a length-of-Britain triathlon by paddleboarding from Land's End to John o' Groats, after having already cycled and walked the route – and asked her for her favourite spot. Her reply: definitely Loch Ness.

Before I left for Scotland, I arranged a sunset SUP with Donald Macpherson, founder of Explore Highland and author of *Great Glen*

Canoe Trail. Who would be more perfect for a guided tour from Dochgarroch Lock to Loch Ness's northern shore at Lochend?

My day is spent at Fort Augustus, a bustling village at the south-west end of Loch Ness, which, with its staircase of five locks and the Caledonian Canal Centre, marks the halfway point of the Great Glen Canoe Trail. There I learn about the civil engineer Thomas Telford, who supervised the canal's construction until it was opened in 1822. The canal is now of such importance it is a scheduled monument. It's a joy to chat to one of the lock-keepers, Drew, from Lancashire, about how much he loves his work.

After sitting happily by the shore gazing in wonder at Loch Ness, I walk past a small Pepperpot lighthouse (built in 1840), so called because it resembles a salt or pepper shaker. There are three along the Caledonian Canal – the other two located at Corpach and Gairlochy.

At dusk, with clouds beginning to gather across the skies, Donald, a lovely family and

I launch from Dochgarroch Lock and make our way through Loch Dochfour to Lochend. Paddling together as a group, Donald shares stories of Loch Ness with us. At 37 kilometres long, nearly three kilometres wide and 230 metres deep, it is home to Scotland's only inland RNLI station, just outside Drumnadrochit. The water in the loch is colder than many parts of the UK's coastline and conditions can be almost like the sea, with waves of over three metres.

We pass the remains of an old coal barge and spot friends of Donald's camping on the shore. Paddling the trail by canoe, kayak or paddleboard is a huge accomplishment and I imagine they will sleep well under the stars tonight. A few drops of rain fall and there is a late-summer chill in the air. I feel a sense of anticipation rising as we edge closer to Lochend. We pass the nineteenth-century Bona Lighthouse, built originally as a dwelling and store and subsequently used to guide boats from the expanse of the loch into the narrower canal. It is now stunning holiday accommodation.

Then, suddenly, there it is: Loch Ness. We stop on the pebbled beach to soak up the magic and majesty of such a huge expanse of water; the fading light of the sun behind the clouds, the dark, grey waters stretching into the distance. The privilege of being on the water is one I never take for granted. I take a moment to whisper, 'thank you'. Lights on the boats at Dochgarroch twinkle as we later return to the pontoon and say our goodbyes after an evening together. The faint sound of voices from the tent on the side of the canal drifts across the quiet waters at the lock as I wrap up and head back to Inverness.

The next morning, I return to Dochgarroch Lock for one last look. 'You're back then?' says one of the lock-keepers, smiling. 'Did you enjoy Loch Ness?' I tell her it was magical.

Two paddleboarders, Gemma and Katie, as well as Katie's dog Fudge are setting out on the final stretch of their journey. With just under eight kilometres to go to Inverness, the two teachers have almost completed the Great Glen Canoe Trail.

I think back to the little girls in the canoe with their dad, paddling with such determination. Whatever your age, your company or your craft, paddling on a Scottish loch is an experience which will make special memories. I write in my journal that one day I would like to SUP the Great Glen Canoe Trail. For now, I wish Gemma, Katie and Fudge well and head to my next destination.

Technical Information

```
DISTANCE
LOCH MORLICH 4km round trip.
LOCH NESS 8km round trip.
..............................................................
LAUNCH LOCATION
LOCH MORLICH
ENTRY AND EXIT POINT NH 972097/57.167, -3.702
TURN AROUND POINT NH 975093/57.163, -3.697
LOCH NESS
ENTRY AND EXIT POINT NH 618404/57.433, -4.303
TURN AROUND POINT NH 601377/57.408, -4.330
```

Difficulty
Loch Morlich
Paddleboarding on Loch Morlich requires knowledge of the wind, although a prevailing wind would mean you would be likely to be blown back to the beach. Paddling close to the beach is lovely, and paddling along Abhainn Ruigh-eunachan was sheltered. There are branches to watch out for and a tiny rapid.

There is another car park on the road from Aviemore, where you can launch easily if good conditions allow.

Loch Ness
Paddleboarding on Loch Dochfour and Loch Ness requires knowledge of the wind and

1 A break at the head of Loch Ness **2** The Pepperpot lighthouse at Fort Augustus
3 The Caledonian Canal **4** Paddling on Loch Dochfour

exit points. Paddleboarding along the length of Loch Ness requires detailed planning and experience. I would recommend a tour with a professional guide.

Getting there
Loch Morlich
The nearest railway station is Aviemore, 10.5km from Loch Morlich, which has direct connections to Glasgow, Inverness and Edinburgh. It is also on the Caledonian Sleeper line. Buses between Aviemore and the Cairngorm Mountain ski centre stop 500m from the launch point.

There is a pay-and-display car park by the beach managed by Forestry and Land Scotland (NH 973097/57.167, -3.698), where there are public toilets.

Loch Ness
Inverness is 10.5km from Loch Ness, where there is a railway station on the Caledonian Sleeper line. Buses from Inverness to Fort William stop on the A82, a few hundred metres from the launch point.

Free parking is available in the Scottish Canals car park (NH 618404/57.433, -4.303).

Route information
The Land Reform (Scotland) Act 2003 means that you do not need a licence to paddle on the Great Glen Canoe Trail (more information can be found at *www.canoescotland.org*). However, if you intend to paddle along the trail Scottish Canals recommend that you register with them seven days before you set off, so you have access to (sometimes payable) facilities en route as well as safety information and updates.

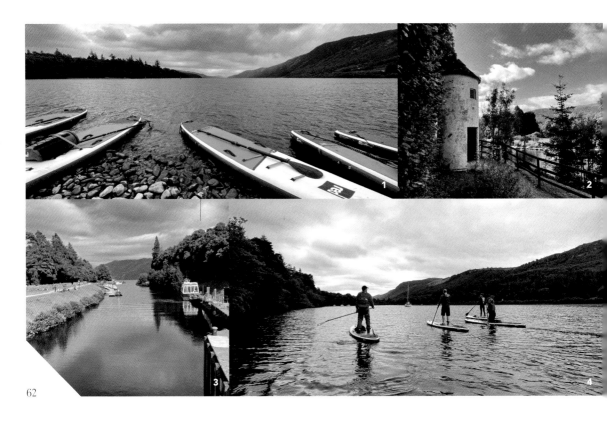

5 Gemma, Katie and Fudge on the Great Glen Canoe Trail

Register at *www.scottishcanals.co.uk* or *www.greatglencanoetrail.info*

Eating and drinking
» Loch Morlich Watersports has the Boathouse Cafe.
» Alternatively, the beach is a lovely place for a picnic.
» An Talla serves breakfast, lunch and cakes.

Instruction, guided tours and equipment hire
» Loch Morlich Watersports has beginner lessons and short guided tours, plus board hire (hardboards).
» Emy McLeod of Strathspey SUP, British Canoeing's Scottish #ShePaddles Ambassador, runs beginner lessons, coaching, guided tours, social SUP events

and board hire in open water, coastal stretches and rivers in the area, including Loch Morlich.
» Donald Macpherson's Explore Highland, based in Inverness, offers bespoke coaching and guided activities throughout the Scottish Highlands.

Further information
» Donald Macpherson, *Great Glen Canoe Trail: A complete guide to Scotland's first formal canoe trail* (Pesda Press, 2011).
» Great Glen Canoe Trail: *www.greatglencanoetrail.info*

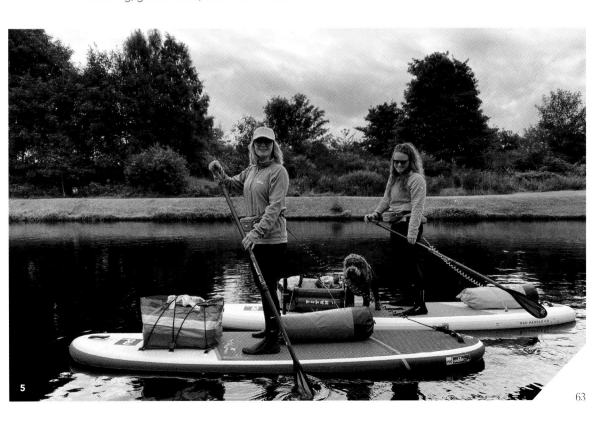

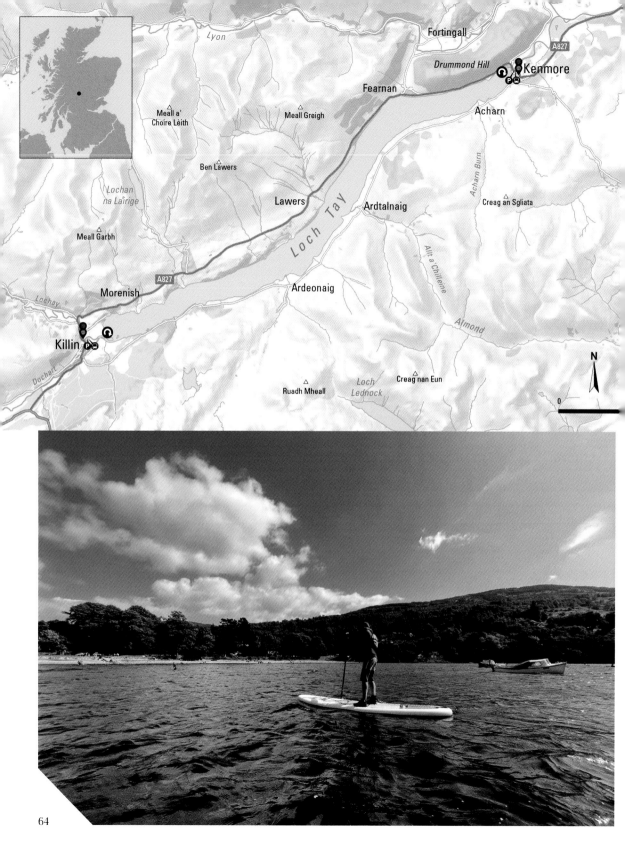

Kenmore and Killin, Loch Tay

SCOTTISH CRANNOGS, FALLING INTO THE SILKY WATERS AND A PICNIC AT DUSK

One of the joys I have experienced time and again while researching this book is the kindness of the paddleboarding community: wisdom, local knowledge and company have been shared so generously. A SUP surfer who embodies this spirit is Matt Gambles, owner of Paddle Surf Scotland and author of *Scottish SUP Guide* and *The SUP Book*. Originally from Yorkshire, Matt has worked in the outdoor industry around the world for over 20 years, taking up paddleboarding in 2009 and launching his business in 2013. He has been a raft guide, bungee-jump master and white water kayaker, and has reached the podium in SUP surf competitions.

We meet on a sunny Monday afternoon in the pretty village of Kenmore on the north-eastern edge of Loch Tay in Perthshire. The car park near the beach is full and I am pumping my board in the square just along from the Kenmore Hotel. Established in 1572, it is thought to be the oldest hotel in Scotland, and Queen Victoria and Prince Albert spent part of their honeymoon here. Robert Burns also visited, writing a poem on the wall that can still be seen today. To my left is the parish church and to my right the gates of Taymouth Castle.

'Hi, Jo, great to meet you,' Matt says, bounding up to me with irrepressible enthusiasm, in his board shorts, Breeze T-shirt and baseball cap. It's just a couple of minutes' walk to the beach, and as we go we chat about conditions. He explains that it's slightly windier than forecast but the southwesterly wind will mean we will be blown back to the shore.

The view across the loch is stunning. At approximately 23 kilometres long, over a kilometre and a half wide and 150 metres at its deepest, Loch Tay is a long, narrow, freshwater loch and is the sixth-largest loch in Scotland. We can see Ben Lawers, the tenth highest Munro in Scotland, set within a National Nature Reserve. The beach, which is sandy and pebbly in parts, slopes gently and children are playing in the waves. There are picnic tables with a special barbecue plate for safety on the grass. There is a joyful, family feel about Kenmore.

We launch from the beach into the breezy sunshine. Our destination is Eilean nam Bannaomh (the Isle of Holy Women), the largest of the 18 crannogs on Loch Tay, lying around 500 metres from the shore. To our left is the Scottish Crannog Centre, a living-history museum documenting life on these Iron Age islands, which were either completely or partially man-made and provided safe settlement for households and animals.

'Team Yorkshire on Loch Tay!' Matt says cheerily as we set off. 'Let's go.'

I follow Matt across the water. Keeping myself upright takes all my concentration as the wind is indeed quite strong. Self-doubt begins to creep in, but Matt is there sharing tips and encouragement. 'Look at the water, read the waves,' he says. 'Keep your head up, you're smashing it.' I might normally have dropped to my knees at this point to lessen the impact of the wind – standing up you are in effect a sail – however, I am taking the opportunity with Matt by my side to improve my technical skills.

We are soon at the island, where we pull up our boards and go exploring. There is something magical about it as we imagine the history and stories it holds. Sybilla of Normandy, the wife of Alexander I and daughter of Henry I of England and his mistress Lady Sybilla Corbet

Opposite Matt paddling at Kenmore

of Alcester, died here in July 1122. A priory dedicated to her memory was built. Around 1474, Sir Colin Campbell built a rampart around the island, making it a fortified residence. Walled remains of both the priory and rampart, plus a well, can still be seen among the lush, green trees.

Back on the water, Matt encourages me to practise my step back turns and I soon find myself in the warm, silky waters of the loch. Laughing, I climb back on my board and we head to Kenmore Bridge, where the loch flows into the mighty River Tay, the longest river in Scotland. Designed by architect John Baxter and completed in 1774, the arches of the bridge create a beautiful, curved outline.

I feel exhilarated and grateful as we arrive back on the beach. Matt zips off to St Andrews for a SUP surf while I enjoy a delicious strawberry ice cream from The Paper Boat on Loch Tay. The owner, Alex, tells me he paddleboarded to work that day – what a wonderful commute. A family are playing with their dog nearby and share stories of their winter paddles to the island, with a flask of hot chocolate to keep them warm. It sounds blissful.

Later that evening, I feel a little restless and decide there is just enough time for a short, safe, solo paddle and picnic from Killin, at the southern end of Loch Tay, near the famous Falls of Dochart. I launch by the Killin Hotel on to the River Lochay and paddle towards the loch. Passing under some bridges, with the leaves gently fluttering in the breeze, the river gradually widens, twisting and turning to the head of the loch. A couple are walking their

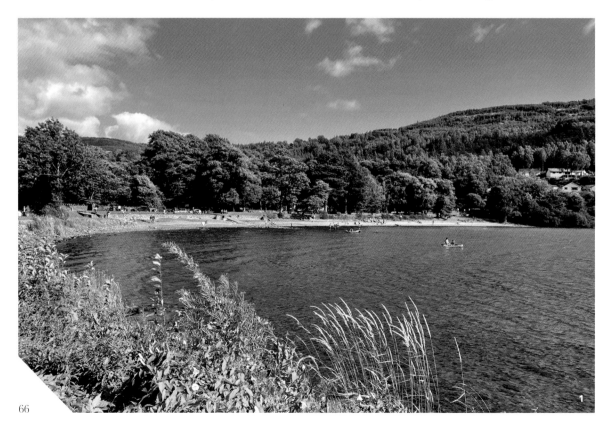

dog, but otherwise I am alone with the swans and the stunning, slightly misty and eerily quiet view ahead. There's a late-summer nip in the air and I turn back, being careful to navigate the shallower waters, returning to the lights and laughter of the hotel at dusk.

It feels a huge privilege to have paddled at both ends of Loch Tay in one day and I begin to imagine what it might feel like, with careful planning, to SUP the length of the loch in its entirety. In 2019 one of Matt's friends, Steve Balfour, paddleboarded from Killin to Kenmore and then from the River Tay to Tayport on the coast, a journey of 210 kilometres, raising money for Parkinson's UK in memory of his grandfather. What an achievement.

I have experienced the wild grace of the loch in all its summer beauty, from the views to Ben Lawers to the wind in my hair and the warm waters I fell in. I imagine as autumn comes and the trees change colour, the days are shorter and the snow arrives on the mountains, you would feel and experience something different. I hope you get chance to enjoy the loch too.

Technical information

DISTANCE
KENMORE **2.5km round trip.**
KILLIN **5km round trip.**

LAUNCH LOCATION
KENMORE
ENTRY AND EXIT POINT **NN 775453/56.583, -3.996**
TURN AROUND POINT **NN 767454/56.584, -4.008**
KILLIN
ENTRY AND EXIT POINT **NN 572333/56.470, -4.319**
TURN AROUND POINT **NN 584336/56.473, -4.299**

ALTERNATIVE ROUTE **My Kenmore route was a short paddle due to the winds but in the right conditions you could enjoy a longer paddle to and around Eilean nam Ban-naomh and along Loch Tay to Fearnan and Acharn.**

Difficulty
Kenmore
An understanding of the wind is important. In flat conditions, the paddle to the island and along the shore would be super. I would recommend a tour guide if you want to SUP on the River Tay for the first time.

Killin
This is a gentle paddle that widens out on to the river, round an island and then to the head of the loch. It is shallow in parts so be aware of your fin. A lovely paddle.

Getting there
Kenmore
The closest railway station is Dunkeld and Birnam, around 34km away, with direct connections to Dumfries and Girvan. A bus, operated by Sweeney's Garage, runs from Aberfeldy. It would be best to check in advance as it does not run on the weekends and only at certain times midweek.

Kenmore is easily reached by car on the A827. There is a small, pay-and-display car park near the beach and by your launch point (NN 773454/56.584, -3.997), but note there is a height limit for vans. Parking fees go to Kenmore in Bloom. There are a small number of free parking spaces in the village and Aberfeldy Road by the beach.

Killin
There are buses (more in the summer) which travel to Callander and stop just by the car park. Killin has Citylink connections to Edinburgh, Glasgow, Inverness, Stirling and Perth.

Killin is easily reached by car along the A827. There is a car park just by McLaren Hall (NN 573332/56.469, -4.318).

1 A post-SUP treat   **2** The famous Falls of Dochart
3 A dusk paddle at Killin

Route information

In Killin, launch by the slip near the Killin Hotel. I gave a donation to the local anglers' club at the Killin Outdoor Centre and Mountain Shop.

Eating and drinking

» The Paper Boat on Loch Tay, owned by Alex and Bridget Martin, is right by the loch. The cafe was closed the day I visited but the ice cream hatch was open and it was delicious.
» The Kenmore Hotel is a short walk from the launch point in Kenmore.
» Mains of Taymouth Courtyard is a 900m walk from the launch point in Kenmore and has a deli and cafe as part of the Mains of Taymouth estate.
» The Killin Hotel is right next to the River Lochay.

Instruction, guided tours and equipment hire

» Matt Gambles's Paddle Surf Scotland offers lessons and equipment hire in the area as well as courses in white water SUP and SUP yoga.

» Unique Adventure Tours Scotland, based in Aberfeldy, runs half-day and full-day SUP expeditions and guided tours.
» Beyond Adventure, based in Aberfeldy, hires paddleboards and also runs SUP tours and microadventures on Loch Tay and surrounding areas.
» Taymouth Marina at the Kenmore end of the loch rents paddleboards.

Further information

» Matt Gambles, *Scottish SUP Guide: Where to stand up paddleboard in Scotland* (self-published, 2020) and *The SUP Book: How to stand up paddleboard* (self-published, 2020).
» At the Scottish Crannog Centre you can find out more about the history of crannogs, the museum and experience hands-on demonstrations: *www.crannog.co.uk*

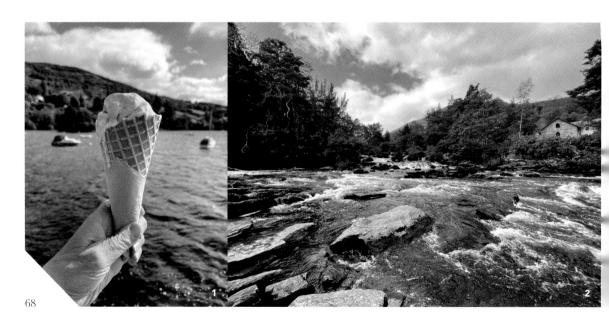

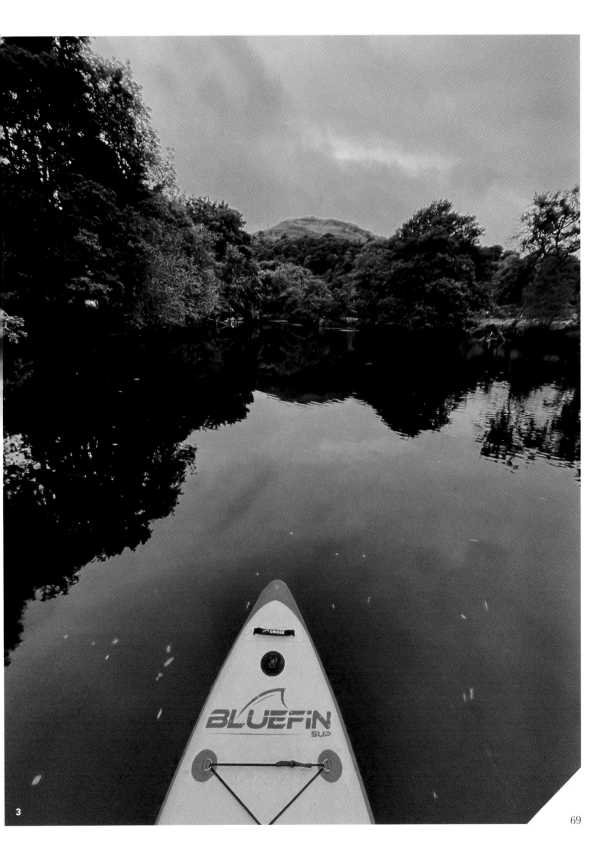

3

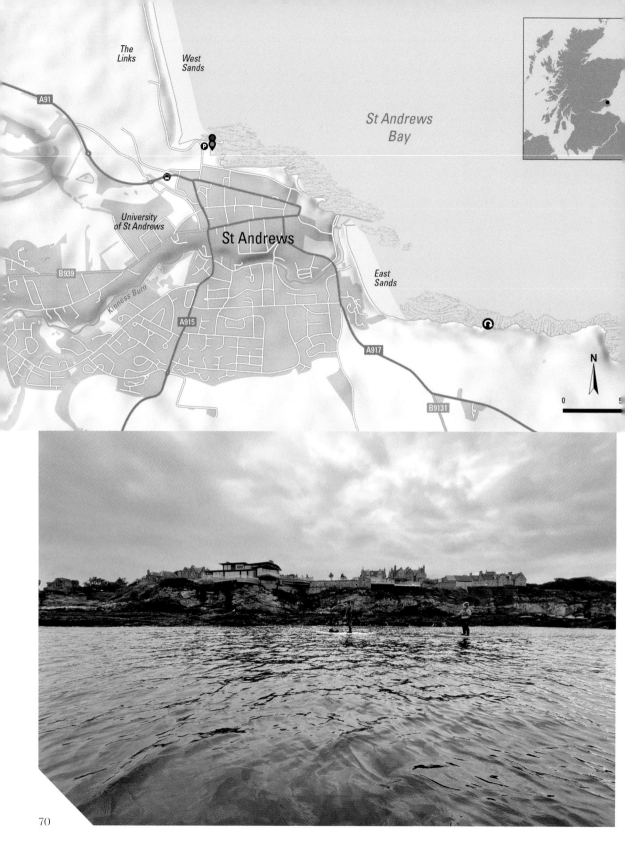

St Andrews and the East Neuk of Fife

FISHING HARBOURS, A CASTLE AND CATHEDRAL, BEAUTIFUL BIRDLIFE AND FLAPJACK ON THE BEACH

'Morning! I slept in a wee bit as we had a shout through the night. I'll be there for half eleven-ish!' a message pings on my phone.

'Super!' I reply. 'I'm just walking from the beach. See you soon!'

It's a sunny Saturday morning in St Andrews, the beautiful Scottish seaside and university town on the east coast of Fife approximately 80 kilometres north-east of Edinburgh, and I am on my way to meet Emily Hague. While I was sleeping soundly at my B & B in Kingsbarns she was out on the sea as volunteer crew with Anstruther RNLI. As well as being a marine biologist and founder of the On the Killer Whale Trail project, Emily also writes about her fascinating adventures with her partner Paul as they hike, camp and spot marine life from Scotland's coastal paths. We both share a love of orcas and the fact that we studied at the University of St Andrews, albeit almost three decades apart.

Sitting in the sunshine at Northpoint Cafe drinking tea, we chat about buoyancy aids, the importance of understanding the wind direction on East Neuk's south-facing coastline and why I have chosen to include the East Neuk in my research (the opportunity to paddleboard in different spots in close proximity). The East Neuk, with *neuk* being the old Scots word for corner or nook, is the area around the eastern peninsula of Fife and south of St Andrews, including the coastal villages and pretty fishing harbours of Crail, Anstruther, Pittenweem, St Monans and Elie.

While Emily returns to Anstruther for a RNLI training exercise, I set about exploring. Emily and Paul (who is a volunteer coastguard) have chosen a route from Elie to Shell Bay and then back to the harbour for our Sunday-morning SUP. We will be following the Fife Coastal Path and Elie Chain Walk route, passing along the sandy Earlsferry and Elie beaches.

After spending the afternoon researching, here are details of three other SUP spots I came across which I think you would enjoy, if wind and tide permits. Crail is a picturesque village with cobbled streets winding down to the small harbour. There's also the seasonal Crail Museum, Crail Pottery and Crail Harbour Gallery and Tea Room. To launch there is a slipway by the harbour to the beach, just down from the picturesque Lobster Cottage. Anstruther has a RNLI station, a lighthouse, an award-winning fish and chip shop and, in the summer, boat trips to the Isle of May to see the puffins. You can launch on the small beach by the RNLI station and stay within the more sheltered harbour. There is also St Monans, which has an unusual zigzag pier, East Pier Smokehouse, the remains of Newark Castle, spectacular views from the church and the beautiful St Monans Windmill near the tidal pool. Look for the Welly Boot Garden and launch from the slip.

The forecast for Sunday is sunshine and a light breeze, and we arrange to meet at 9.a.m. in the car park by the Harbour Cafe, run by Jack and Amy Elles who appeared on BBC Two's *Great British Menu*. When Sunday arrives, however, the weather has different ideas: it is grey and blustery and the sea is beginning to look choppy. It is definitely do-able but doesn't exactly look like the joyful paddle and picnic

Opposite Paddling around St Andrews

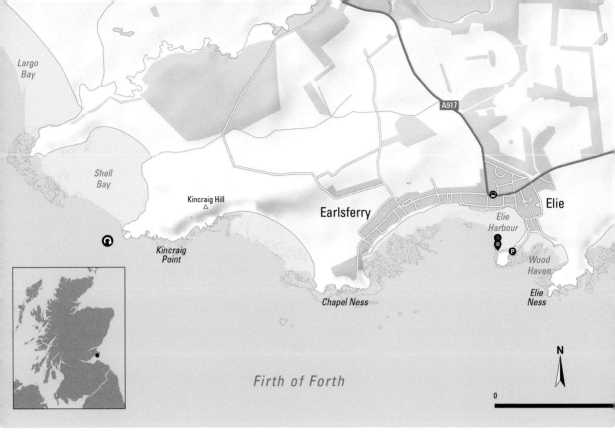

Largo
Bay

Shell
Bay

Kincraig Hill
△

Kincraig
Point

Earlsferry

Elie
Harbour

Elie

Wood
Haven

Chapel Ness

Elie
Ness

A917

N

Firth of Forth

0

we had planned. Emily's mum has even sent her homemade flapjack from Yorkshire for the occasion! We check the weather along the coast and within a couple of minutes Paul's mum has confirmed that there is barely a whisper of wind in St Andrews.

Grateful to have a plan B, we leave for St Andrews about 21 kilometres away, and are soon parked by the R&A World Golf Museum. With the smartest public toilets I've ever changed in and just a few steps away from the beach, it is an ideal spot to pump up our boards and launch. Behind us is RNLI-lifeguarded St Andrews West Sands, almost three kilometres of sandy beach famous for being featured in the opening scene of *Chariots of Fire*. Ahead is East Sands as well as the ruins of St Andrews Cathedral, founded in 1160 and consecrated in July 1318. We will also pass the pier where students of the University of St Andrews, in their distinctive red gowns, walk on a Sunday

morning after chapel and at the beginning of the academic year – this is known as the Pier Walk. Another tradition is 'The Gaudie' on 30 April, a procession by candlelight, led by a piper, to leave a wreath at the site of a shipwreck. This is to commemorate the courage of former student John Honey, who on 3 January 1800 single-handedly rescued five men from the wreck of *Janet* of Macduff, which had run aground on East Sands.

We set off along the cliffs, taking in the magnificent history along the way. As we paddle towards Kinkell Braes, near the sea stack called Maiden's Rock, we chat about a local Facebook group, Forth Marine Mammals, where sightings of dolphins, seals, whales and other marine life are shared. I've since joined and it is an inspiring read if you ever need a dose of coastal joy.

Today it is the birds keeping us company, providing the soundtrack to our easy paddling; fulmars, kittiwake, razor bills, guillemots and

Opposite The beautiful water at St Andrews © Paul Hutchison, @onthekillerwhaletrail

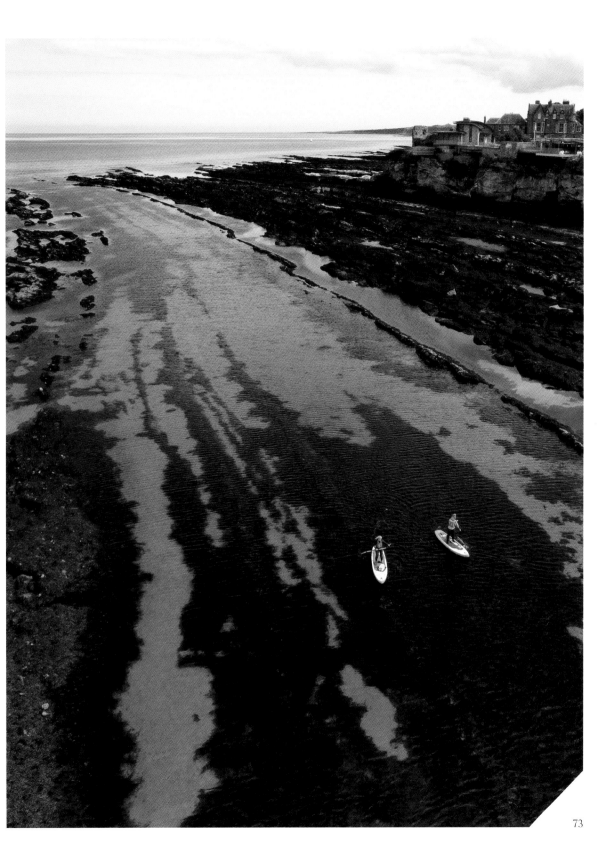

1 Paul paddling at Kinkell Braes   **2** Paul and Emily, with St Andrews in the distance

oystercatchers swooping, swimming and diving into the sea. I'm glad of Emily and Paul's ornithological expertise.

After about an hour we reach the rocks, carefully pull up our boards and find a spot to enjoy Mrs Hague's flapjack and a cup of tea. The sun beats down on our backs and the morning's grey skies have turned to blue. I'm pleased I have brought my mask and snorkel as once we are on the water again we spend half an hour looking into the rock pools from our boards, marvelling at the crabs and different types of seaweed. Gradually we make our way back, listening to the birds, spotting fish and appreciating the historic views ahead.

It wasn't the paddleboarding and picnic we had planned, and yet it seemed almost like it was meant to be. An easy Sunday morning nourishing the soul in a town that means so much to all of us. I can only imagine how full your sense of wonder and adventure would be after a week in this area, exploring the villages and harbours on this coastline. They are all on my wish list for another year. I also make a note to read more about identifying birds and seaweed; there's always something to learn when we step on a paddleboard.

A #2MinuteBeachClean, one last walk to the Quad and it's time to leave St Andrews and head to my next destination. I have sand between my toes and a full and very grateful heart.

Technical information

DISTANCE
ST ANDREWS **6.25km round trip.**
ELIE **9km round trip.**

....

LAUNCH LOCATION
ST ANDREWS
ENTRY AND EXIT POINT **NO 506172/56.345, -2.802**
TURN AROUND POINT **NO 528158/56.332, -2.766**
ELIE
ENTRY AND EXIT POINT **NT 492996/56.186, -2.820**
TURN AROUND POINT **NT 460997/56.186, -2.871**

Difficulty

Paddleboarding experience is necessary for this trip and knowledge of wind and tides is important. Paddleboarding close to our launch point and hugging the cliff is more sheltered. St Andrews West Sands and East Sands are suited to SUP surfing.

Getting there
St Andrews

St Andrews is well connected by rail, bus and car. By railway, you could arrive at Leuchars

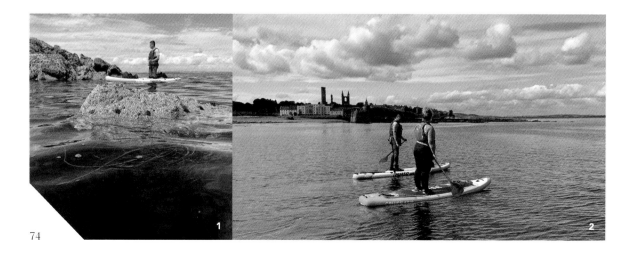

3 Emily and Paul with St Andrew's Cathedral in the background
Overleaf Great Cumbrae from Largs, the Cumbraes © Shutterstock/Victoria Boyce

station and then take a taxi or the frequent bus between St Andrews and Dundee. From the bus station, St Andrews West Sands is just over a kilometre away.

We parked at the pay-and-display Bruce Embankment car park on Golf Place (NO 506172/ 56.344, -2.801), and launched at the beach just in front. There are paid public toilets in the car park.

Elie
Buses to Leven, Edinburgh and St Andrews stop on the High Street in Elie, 800m from the launch point. There is a pay-and-display car park, which has public toilets, along The Toft by the harbour and near Elie Watersports (NT 493996/56.186, -2.818).

Route information
There are RNLI lifeguards at St Andrews West Sands and East Sands and Elie in the summer.

Eating and drinking
» There are lots of lovely cafes in St Andrews. We had a delicious brunch at Northpoint Cafe on North Street.
» The Cheesy Toast Shack on the East Sands serves toasties and hot drinks.

» Jannettas Gelateria, which also serves breakfast, ciabattas and cakes, is a well-known landmark on South Street and has been serving ice cream for over 110 years.
» The Harbour Cafe is by the car park in Elie and open during the summer.
» The Ship Inn is a pub along The Toft which is open all day for food and drinks.

Instruction, guided tours and equipment hire
» Blown Away offers SUP safaris in St Andrews, including hot chocolate and shortbread.
» Och Aye Canoe offers paddleboarding lessons for beginners and advanced skills at Lochore Meadows, about 45km inland from St Andrews.
» Elie Watersports offers SUP hire and lessons.

Further information
» On the Killer Whale Trail: *www.onthekillerwhaletrail.com*

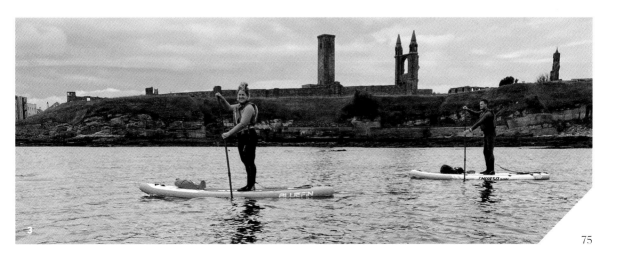

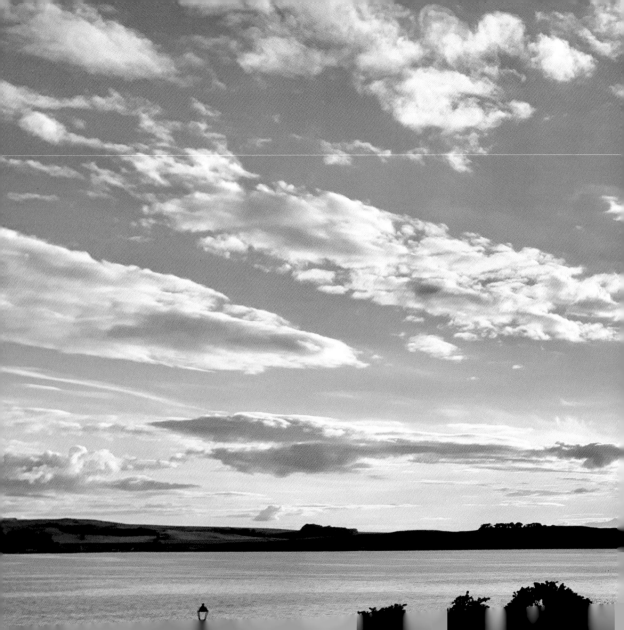

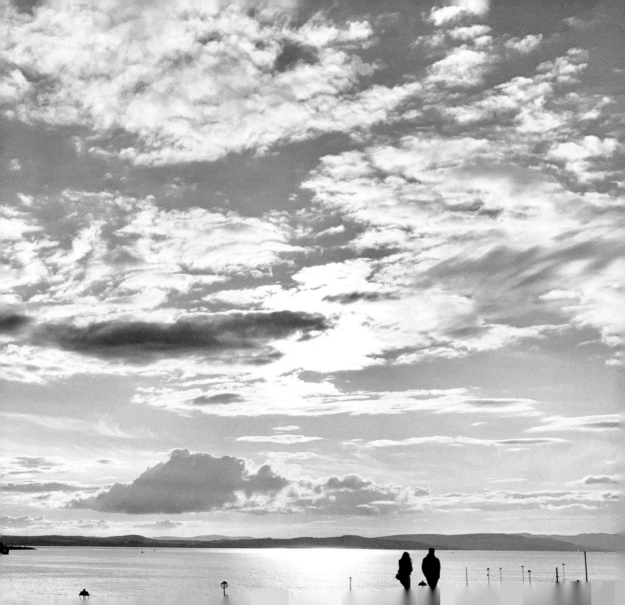

'Possibilities, big horizons, tiny details … all the possibilities of paddleboarding.'

These were my scribbled notes as I planned my travels. The Lake District offered iconic mountain views on Derwent Water (p203) and Ullswater (p197). Cornwall brought dramatic cliffs on the Lizard peninsula (p149), The Gannel's turquoise waters (p167) and paddleboarding picnics in Porthpean (p161). Sidmouth offered glassy waters (p131), Lympstone a sunset show (p137) and Salcombe Harbour beautiful creeks (p143). Old Harry Rocks was an early morning adventure (p125).

Liverpool (p185) showed me how unique SUP in the city can be. Cullercoats on the north-east coast gifted a stunning lighthouse (p83). Runswick Bay in Yorkshire allowed me to share a childhood gem (p89). In Wells-next-the-Sea in Norfolk, salt marsh creeks filled the soul (p101).

Canals provided a lesson in history, including London's Regent's Canal (p107), the Leeds and Liverpool Canal (p191), the Kennet and Avon near Bath (p173), Nottingham's Beeston Canal (p95) as well as the Exeter Ship Canal (p137) and the Royal Military Canal in Kent (p119).

Rivers allowed me to whoosh along the River Trent (p95), spot otters on the River Severn (p179) and experience the tidal River Exe (p137), as well as the River Fowey (p155) and the River Thames (p113).

To travel as my scribbled notes became a reality was an honour. I hope they serve as a useful guide as you explore the magic on our doorsteps.

ENGLAND

Opposite Paddling on Ullswater   **Overleaf** Taking in the view of Runswick Bay © Charlotte Graham

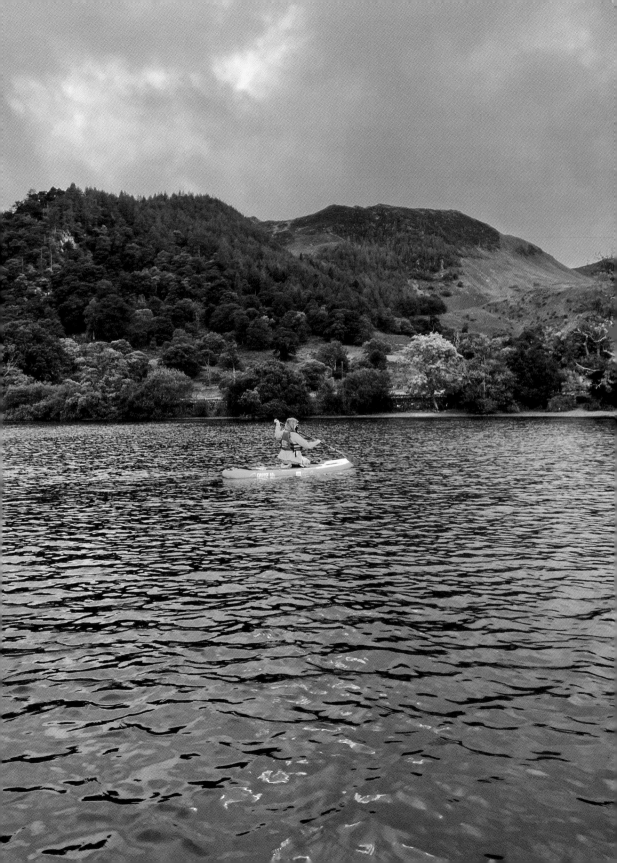

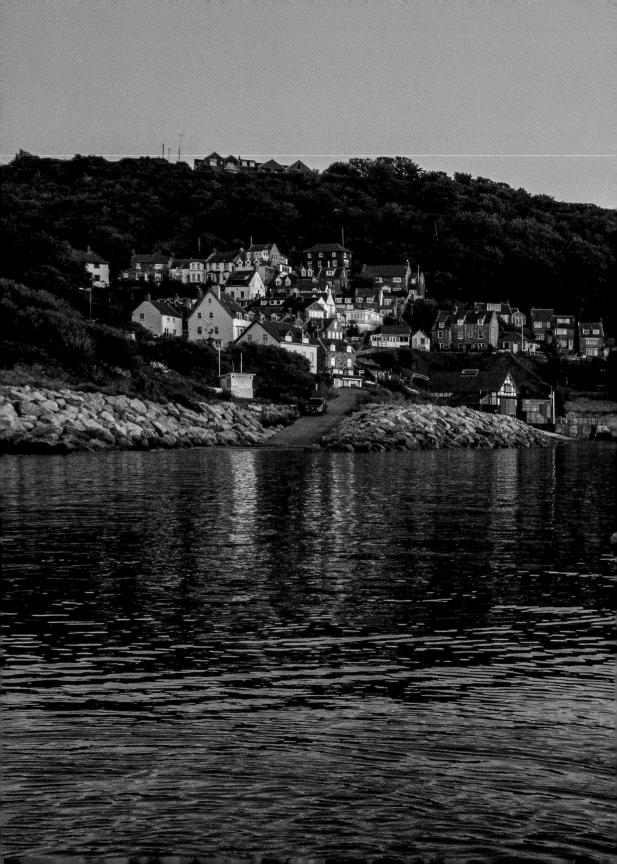

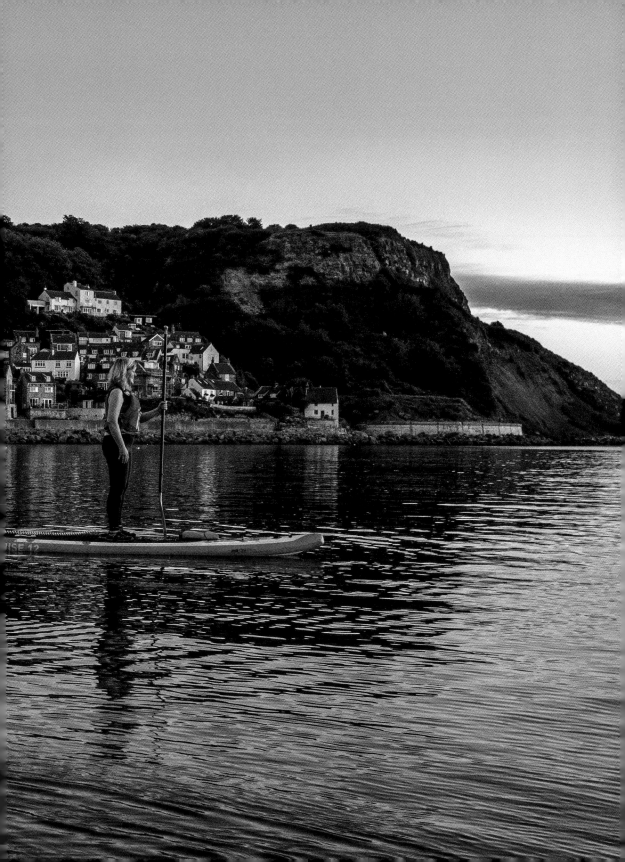

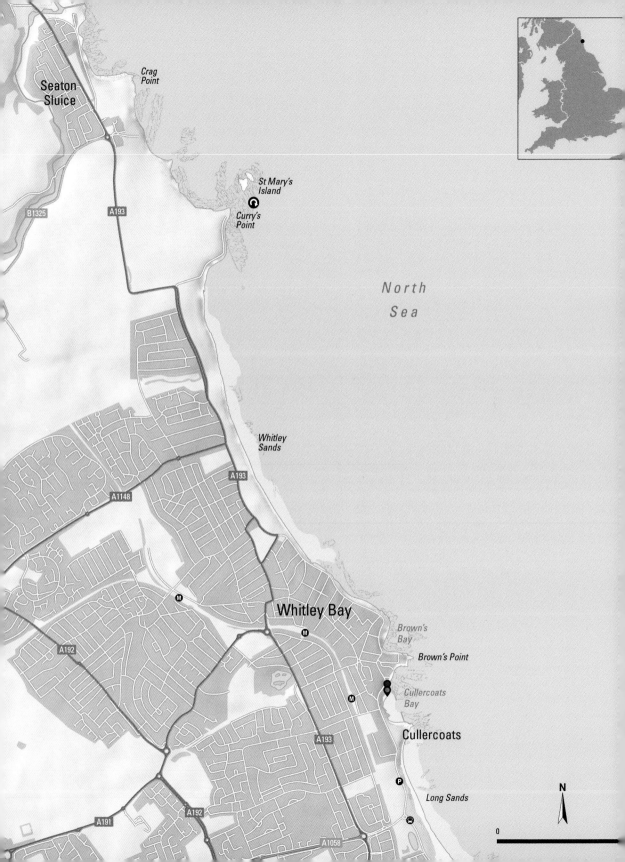

Seaton
Sluice

Crag
Point

*St Mary's
Island*

*Curry's
Point*

B1325

A193

*North
Sea*

*Whitley
Sands*

A193

A1148

M

Whitley Bay

M

*Brown's
Bay*

Brown's Point

A192

M

*Cullercoats
Bay*

Cullercoats

A193

P

Long Sands

A192

A191

A1058

N

0

Cullercoats Bay to St Mary's Lighthouse

GRACE DARLING, AN INQUISITIVE SEAL, RNLI HISTORY AND PADDLING THROUGH THE CAVES

'You do know the sun always shines in the North East?' Heather says, smiling, as we sit drinking tea planning our afternoon on the sea.

'Of course,' I reply, reflecting upon how lucky we are that the strong offshore winds forecast earlier in the week have not materialised. There are blue skies above and we have a lovely weather window to paddleboard from Cullercoats Bay to St Mary's Lighthouse in Whitley Bay and back.

I am here with Heather Peacock, SUP surfer, sea swimmer and mum of two, who combines teaching paddleboarding with working for the charity Children's Cancer North. Her first SUP experience was in Maui in 2007. With a signed picture of big-wave surfer Laird Hamilton and a wooden paddle in her hallway, Heather is definitely one of the UK's paddleboarding pioneers.

Bringing my board Grace to the North East to paddle to a lighthouse feels extra special. She is named after Grace Darling, the RNLI heroine, who lived with her family at Longstone Lighthouse off the Northumberland coast. On 7 September 1838 Grace rescued survivors of the steamship SS *Forfarshire* that had run aground on the Farne Islands. Aged just 22, she was awarded the RNLI's Silver Medal for Gallantry. The beautiful RNLI Grace Darling Museum in Bamburgh, approximately 80 kilometres north of Cullercoats, is well worth a visit.

Nestled between Tynemouth's King Edward's Bay, Long Sands to the south and Whitley Bay to the north, Cullercoats is a village on the North Tyneside coastline. The bay has a sandy beach with two small piers and is a sheltered spot for families and water-sports fans. The harbour has a rich fishing heritage and previously had coal- and salt-shipping industries, and there are still the small fishing boats known as cobles in the bay. It has also attracted artists, among them the American Winslow Homer, who lived here from 1881 to 1882. According to the Metropolitan Museum of Art in New York, Homer, 'became sensitive to the strenuous and courageous lives of its inhabitants, particularly the women, whom he depicted hauling and cleaning fish, mending nets, and, most poignantly, standing at the water's edge, awaiting the return of their men. When the artist returned to New York, both he and his art were greatly changed.'

Today Cullercoats has a thriving cafe culture and in the bay there is the Dove Marine Laboratory, part of Newcastle University's School of Marine Science and Technology, a #2MinuteBeachClean board and a RNLI station. In 2021, Anna Heslop became the station's first female helm in its 170-year history.

The beach has a lovely, friendly feel to it and as we arrive there are children building sandcastles as well as swimmers and paddleboarders enjoying the harbour under the watchful eye of the RNLI lifeguards. We make our way out to sea, heading to Whitley Bay round an outcrop of rocks on the headland, where we later watch a chap enjoying some coasteering. To the south we can see Tynemouth Priory and Castle as well as Tynemouth Pier and Lighthouse.

What strikes me first is the clarity of the water as we paddle over rock pools and watch

1 Paddling past Whitley Bay   **2** Heading towards the caves near Cullercoats

the seaweed swaying in the waves. The sea is glassy, and it is a lovely 90-minute paddle for five kilometres to St Mary's Lighthouse. We chat about the tides, the kindness of the SUP community and Cullercoats Collective, a community interest company which has the aim to promote the village as a great place to live, work and play. We spot lion's mane jellyfish and Heather sees a plaice swim past. Standing on a paddleboard always gives such a great opportunity to see what's beneath the waves.

As we reach St Mary's the afternoon sun casts a beautiful glow over the tower. The lighthouse was completed in 1898 and operated until 1984. With the former keeper's cottage, it is now a visitor centre and shop – you can climb the 137 steps should you wish to. The tiny island is also surrounded by a nature reserve

with rock pools, clifftop grassland and man-made wetland habitats.

As we gently bob along on our boards, being careful to not get close to the island as it is a haul-out site for seals, I realise we are not alone: there are cormorants on a nearby rock and two seals playing and diving around us. To my right I glimpse a seal that's turned on its back and is gently floating under my board, almost as if it wants me to scratch its stomach. Instead of fumbling for a photo, I simply watch and soak up this tiny moment of wonder. My friend Dr Sarah Perkins later tells me it was probably a young seal being inquisitive.

Before heading back we stop briefly to chat to an angler in his kayak, enjoying the sun. En route, the wind picks up from the south and we paddle with gusto, keeping closer to the

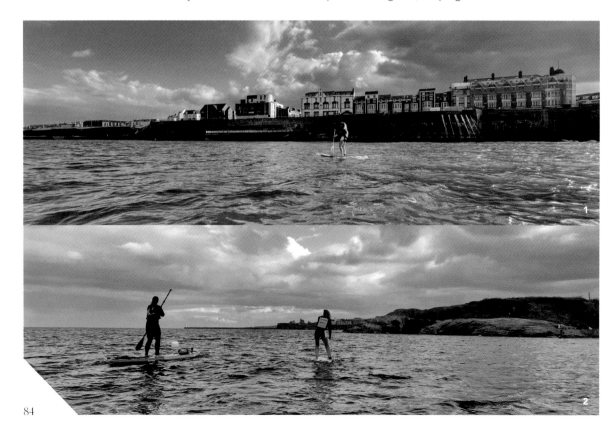

3 Reaching St Mary's Lighthouse

shore for safety and shelter. At the edge of the harbour, we meet a local paddler and invite her to join us as we have fun paddleboarding through the caves now the tide is up. The cooing of a pigeon perched on a rock in the cave and the splash of waves add a final noisy finish to our adventure.

It's early evening and the bay has a jolly, summery feel. Young people are laughing and jumping into the sea from the pier. There are dippers, swimmers, paddlers and beach cleaners. Among them is Katie Atherton, director of the Cullercoats Collective which Heather had mentioned. She tells me about the 'trash mob' text-alert system they have set up, with over 200 volunteers who will come to the beach to pick litter at short notice to save any plastic entering the sea. They also held a

children's beach Olympics. From everything I have experienced, their focus on creating their goals of pride in place, a warm welcome and celebration of Cullercoats is working a treat: Grace and I have had a gorgeous day here.

As I leave the bay I stop to savour the view and soak up the atmosphere one more time before we head to Heather's for pizza with her family. I fall into bed that night happily exhausted and with a full heart, only just managing not to sleep in my swimsuit.

The harbour seemingly had a profound impact on Winslow Homer over a century ago. I think the same has happened to me. Perhaps it will for you too.

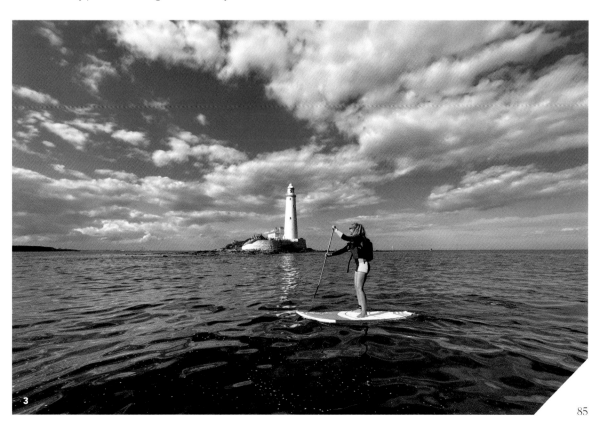

Technical information

DISTANCE **10km round trip.**

....

LAUNCH LOCATION
ENTRY AND EXIT POINT **NZ 364713/55.0349, -1.432**
TURN AROUND POINT **NZ 353752/55.068, -1.448**

....

ALTERNATIVE ROUTE **You can also reach St Mary's Lighthouse from Whitley Bay, which is closer.**

Difficulty

Paddleboarding experience is necessary for this trip and knowledge of wind and tides is important for St Mary's Lighthouse if you're going independently.

Cullercoats would be a lovely spot to enjoy close to the beach in the harbour and by the caves at high tide.

Getting there

The nearest railway station is Newcastle upon Tyne, and from here take the Metro's Yellow Line to Cullercoats station. Frequent buses to Gateshead and Whitley Bay stop just across the road from the beach. There are public toilets by the RNLI station.

There is a pay and display at Beaconsfield car park (NZ 365 706/55.029,-1.431). If you park at the north end of the car park, you can access the south side of the beach within 600m.

Route information

There are RNLI lifeguards in the summer at Cullercoats's beach.

The closest Magicseaweed webcams are Tynemouth at Long Sands and Whitley Bay.

Eating and drinking

» There are lots of cafes in Cullercoats. Try Cullercoats Coffee and The Boatyard.

Instruction, guided tours and equipment hire

» CBK Adventures offers lessons, equipment hire, courses and guided tours, including to St Mary's Lighthouse. It is just under a kilometre's walk from Cullercoats Bay. It also offers SUP cookout tours and kayak lessons, tours and hire.

Further information

» Cullercoats Collective: *www.cullercoatscollective.co.uk*
» St Mary's Lighthouse: *www.visitnorthtyneside.com*
» The RNLI Grace Darling Museum: *www.rnli.org.uk*
» 2 Minute Foundation: *www.beachclean.net*

Opposite Exploring the caves near Cullercoats

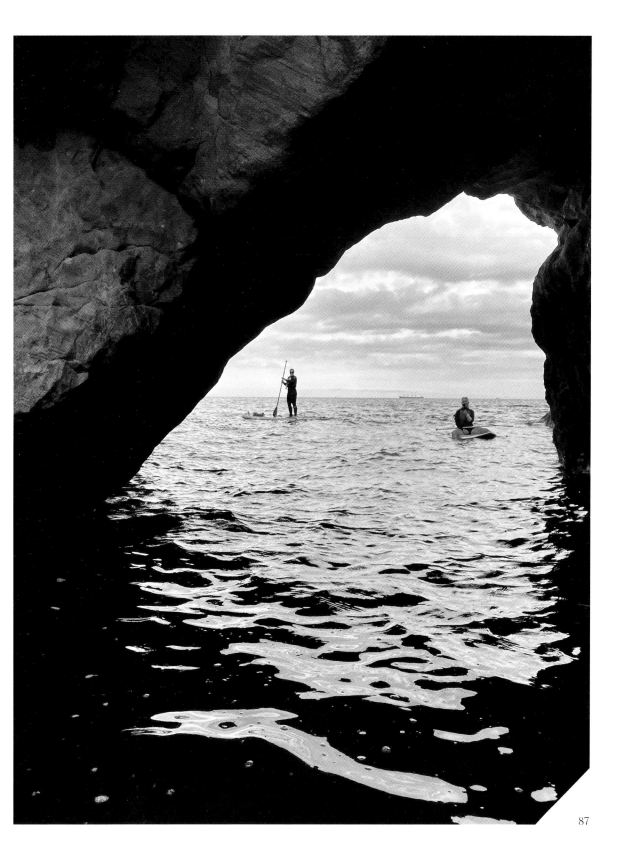

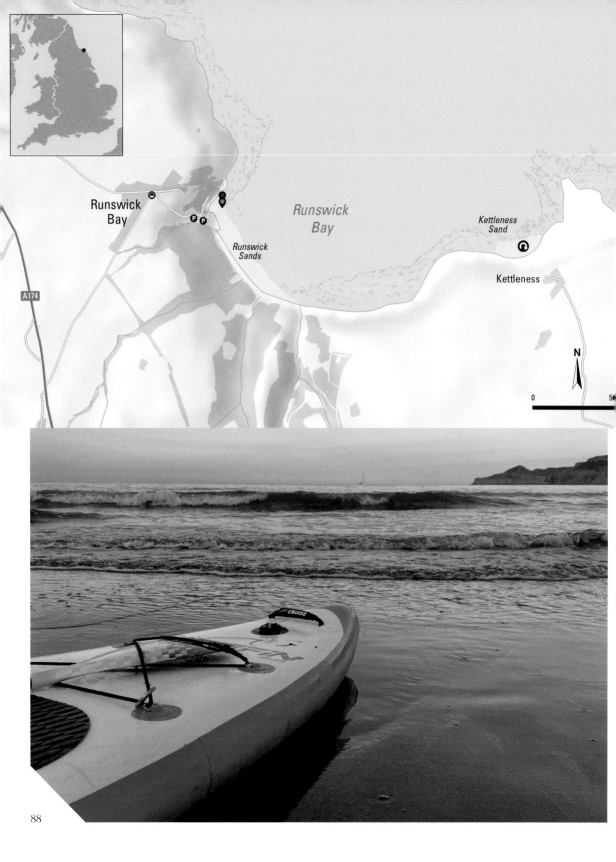

Runswick Bay

Runswick Bay

Runswick Sands

Kettleness Sand

Kettleness

A174

N

0   5

Runswick Bay

**SUNRISE SUP, A HIDDEN GEM, CHILDHOOD
MEMORIES AND RECORD-BREAKING ADVENTURERS
ON THE HORIZON**

'Stop there! Now hold as still as you can. Great. Just a little longer …' says the voice over the walkie talkie. I breathe as calmly as I can, feeling the sea beneath me ever so slightly rise and fall.

'We can do this, Grace,' I whisper to my paddleboard. 'Let's get this right for Charlotte.'

It's 5.15 a.m. on a Saturday morning in August and I am on the North Sea at Runswick Bay on the Yorkshire coast. The light cloud covering has lifted and the sky is now a deep orange as the sun rises over the horizon. The warmth of its glow bathes the red roof tiles of the tiny cottages that cling, higgledy-piggledy, to the cliff. The sailing boat behind us sways and creaks gently on its mooring.

'Got it. Perfect. Now go for a paddle and I'll take some drone footage. Enjoy!'

Exhaling, I follow the light on the water, enjoying the solitude of a soul-nourishing dawn SUP before returning to the beach to chat to award-winning Yorkshire photographer Charlotte Graham. Her brief is to take some sunrise photographs of paddleboarders for a national newspaper. She invited me to meet her on the beach at 4.15 a.m. By 6.15 a.m., she's back up the very steep hill to the bank top and on to her next assignment.

Runswick Bay is a small village about 14.5 kilometres north-west of Whitby and four kilometres south of Staithes. Its sweeping, crescent-shaped beach was the *Times* and *Sunday Times* Best Beach of the Year in 2020 and it's regularly described as a hidden gem by holidaymakers and travel writers.

A white, Grade-II thatched cottage, previously the coastguard's, perches on the northern edge of the village by the old, curved sea wall. This was fortified in 2018 by the rock armour brought in to protect the village from coastal erosion. The rock pools nearby are a great spot for fossil hunting, and a local natural historian offers fossil forage and beach safaris. The former RNLI lifeboat house is now home to the independent Runswick Bay Rescue Boat and sits next to the slip, covered in brightly coloured canoes, kayaks and rowing boats. Sandside Cafe, affectionately known locally as Aunty Pat's, serves ice cream, sandwiches, homemade cakes and tea in proper crockery. One of my favourite summer-holiday jobs was at Sandside Cafe on the sweet counter in 1978 selling 99s, candy necklaces and MoJo chews. On your way to the beach, you'll pass the #2MinuteBeachClean board and the RNLI lifeguard cabin. They are always very happy to talk through weather and sea conditions.

The impressive headland to the east of the bay is Kettleness, the site of a former alum and jet works, and next to the point is a small beach. The cliffs above are part of the Cleveland Way, a 174-kilometre walking trail officially opened in May 1969 which was the second recognised National Trail in England and Wales. It starts inland in the town of Helmsley, passes through the heather moorland of the North York Moors National Park to Saltburn and then Whitby and Robin Hood's Bay, ending in Filey.

The story I've always been told is that in the 1680s almost all of the houses in Runswick Bay, which used to be a thriving fishing village, fell into the sea. Fortunately there were no fatalities as the families were alerted by two mourners at a wake who raised the alarm. Only one home remained standing – it belonged to the gentleman whose funeral they were attending.

Opposite Grace at Runswick Bay

1 A sunny paddle   **2** The thatched cottage at the northern edge of the village
3 Runswick Bay at sunrise   **4** Grace resting on Runswick Bay's beach

Later, in the 1880s, the village was popular with artists such as Frederick William Jackson and Ralph Hedley, who were drawn both by the seascape and hard-working fishing families.

With its views of pretty cottages and easy access, paddleboarding from the smaller of the two Runswick Bay beaches, near the old lifeboat house, is wonderful. An hour either side of high tide, it is a lovely place to build your technical skills and confidence. You can stay close to the shore and yet feel a world away. The previously mentioned Grade-II-listed thatched cottage also acts as a marker if you want to ensure you are not moving too far away from the shore. As your experience grows and with calm conditions, the five-kilometre-round trip to Kettleness is a joyful sea adventure. I've often been joined momentarily by an inquisitive seal and am hopeful one day I'll be on my board when the dolphins visit. There are lion's mane and mauve stinger jellyfish, gannets, guillemots, cormorants and of course seagulls. Give the lobster pots

and cobles (fishing boats) a wide berth and make your way across. If you're lucky, you may see the RNLI Staithes and Runswick Bay lifeboat crew on a training exercise in the bay.

I launch from the beach at Runswick Bay and paddle over to the beach at Kettleness. This little beach has its own waterfall and is a great spot for some SUP snorkelling from your board, watching the kelp and crabs beneath. The waves break powerfully on the point itself so I keep away. It is quite enough to watch them and then look north along the coastline to Port Mulgrave, Staithes and the North East. My dream is to one day paddle the Yorkshire coastline with friends, stopping to beach clean along the way.

While a sunrise SUP is hard to beat, it is also very special when the sun sets behind the village; the light reflecting on Kettleness gives the cliff face a deep-red aura. It was on such an evening in the summer of 2021 that I watched Brendon Prince paddleboard across the bay on

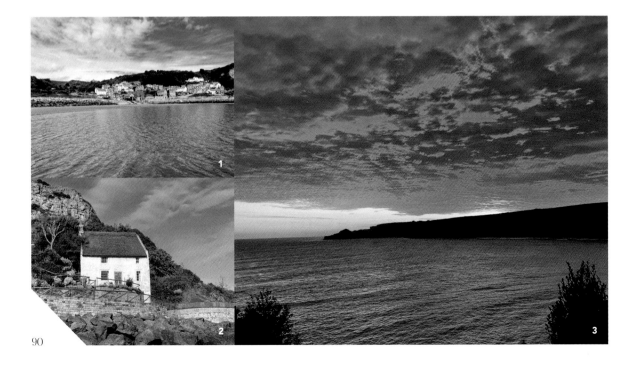

his journey to become the first person to SUP circumnavigate the coastline of mainland Britain in 141 days, raising awareness of water safety and funds for the RNLI, Above Water and The Wave Project.

We all have our own paddleboarding journeys to share: our first lesson, the thrill of standing up or the moment we realise we can walk on water. There are places where we learn how to paddleboard and there are places where we become paddleboarders. Derwent Water is the former for me, Runswick Bay the latter. It is where I fell in love with the possibilities of SUP and gained a new perspective, literally and figuratively, of a village I've known for over 45 years.

The bay is indeed a gem that I treasure every time I set off from the beach and follow my glitter path of joy. I hope to see you there one day.

Technical information

DISTANCE **5km round trip.**
LAUNCH LOCATION ENTRY AND EXIT POINT **NZ 811160/54.532, -0.749** TURN AROUND POINT **NZ 829158/54.530, -0.721**

Difficulty

Paddleboarding experience is necessary for a trip to Kettleness and knowledge of wind and tides is important if going independently. Paddleboarding by the beach is lovely.

Launch by either of the two slipways. The beach is flat and mostly sandy. You may be tempted to launch or exit by the sailing club further along the beach if it is a busy day – I wouldn't recommend this. The beach slopes steeply and you may soon be waist-deep, creating a much more powerful wave to contend with.

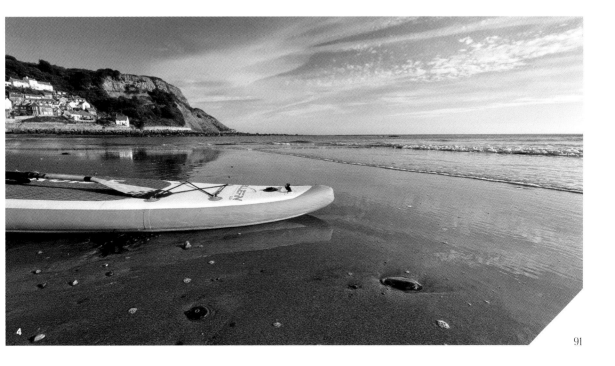

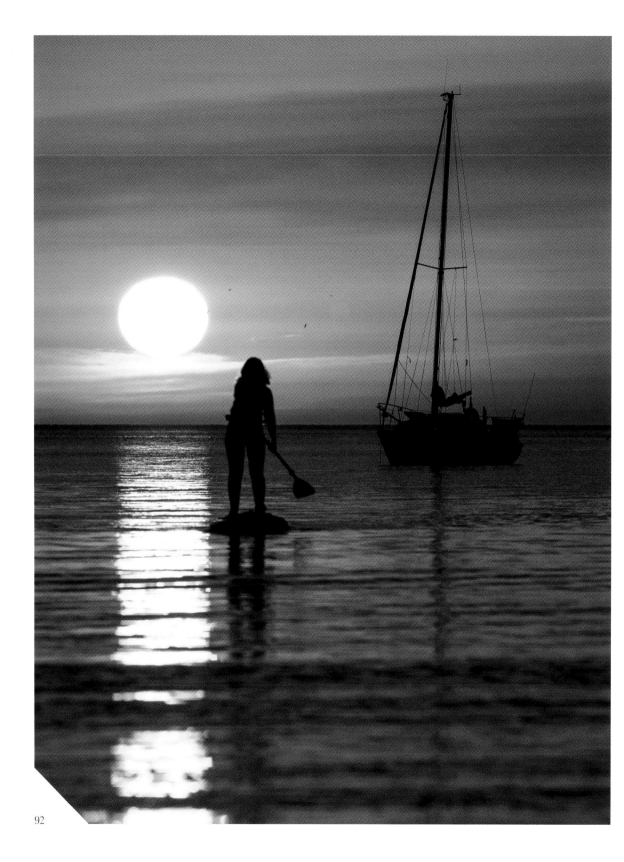

Low tide reveals the rocks along the shoreline. These are wonderful for rock pooling and fossil hunting, however they do make it tricky for paddleboarding through. Be careful of your fin.

The cliffs may protect the beach from the wind, however as you paddle from the shore the wind will be stronger so be aware of conditions. Be aware of the cliffs as there are landslips.

Getting there

A bus from Whitby to Middlesbrough runs regularly to the top of Runswick Bay bank, 500m from the launch point. The closest railway station is Whitby, with direct connections to Newcastle.

You can reach Runswick Bay by car via the A174. There is one steep road into the village, which is a 1:4 gradient. There is a car park a couple of hundred metres from the beach at the bottom of the hill (NZ 809159/54.532, -0.751). This is a pay and display – do bring cash as phone reception is very poor and you are unlikely to get a signal to pay online. I suggest you don't turn north-east at the roundabout as there is no parking in the centre of the village. There is also parking at the top of the bank at very busy times.

Route information

There are RNLI lifeguards at Runswick Bay beach in the summer.

Eating and drinking

» Sandside Cafe is right by the beach. It serves cakes, sandwiches, ice cream and hot drinks. There are public toilets just behind the cafe.
» The Royal Hotel is in the village, just a few hundred metres from the car park.
» Beech Grove Bakery serves delicious artisan bread and cakes.

Instruction, guided tours and equipment hire

» Barefoot Kayak hires out paddleboards and kayaks on the beach in the school summer holidays. Outside of those times, they offer British Canoeing Personal Performance Awards.
» Whitby Surf School offers lessons, board hire and sunrise/sunset paddles in Whitby.
» SUP Adventures runs lessons, guided tours and SUP yoga in Whitby and on the River Esk.

Further information

» Peter McGrath's Runswick fossil forage and shore safari: *www.facebook.com/ Barefootfossilwalks*
» Cleveland Way: *www.nationaltrail.co.uk*
» Fins, Feathers & Fish Wildlife Trips offers dolphin and whale spotting with Sean Baxter on his boat *All My Sons* from Staithes: *www.realstaithes.com*
» Brendon Prince, The Long Paddle: *www.thelongpaddle.co.uk*

Opposite Paddling early enough to catch the sunrise © Charlotte Graham

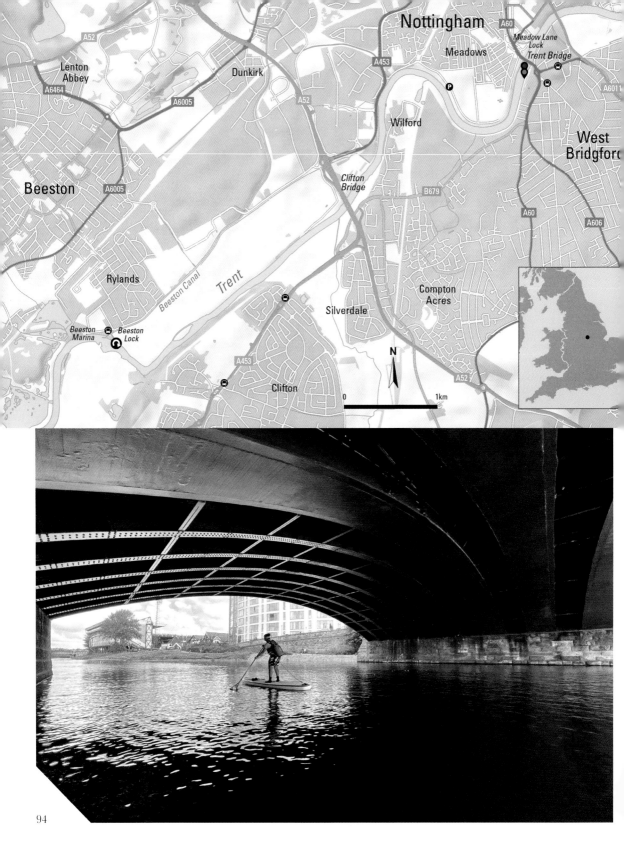

Trent Loop, Nottingham

**RAILWAY ADVENTURES, FINDING THE EXTRA-
ORDINARY IN THE ORDINARY, CANAL HIGH FIVES
WITH STRANGERS AND RIDING THE WATER TRAIN**

'Hey, let's give each other a high five!' says a
jolly woman on a paddleboard approaching
me as we paddle near Castle Wharf on the
Nottingham and Beeston Canal. A little
surprised but happy to say hello, I raise my
hand, and on a sunny Saturday morning in
Nottingham complete strangers briefly share
the joy of an urban SUP together. We wish each
other well and paddle on.

I'm here with my friend Dr Adya Misra,
geneticist, SUP coach, experienced kayaker
and kayak teacher, paddleboarding a slightly
modified version of the Trent Loop Challenge,
one of 35 places Adya has challenged herself
to paddle in one year. Nottingham has been
on my wish list for a long time, recommended
as a favourite spot by Darren and Dale from
the Stand Up Paddle UK community and
family friends who have kayaked through their
home city many times. Like Regent's Canal in
London (p107), Bristol Harbourside (p173) and
Liverpool's Royal Albert Dock (p185), I was keen
to share another launch point that you can
reach by public transport, if you are happy and
able to carry your board on a train or bus.

The Trent Loop is a 22.5-kilometre
circular challenge along the River Trent and
Nottingham and Beeston Canal. It starts and
finishes at Holme Pierrepont Country Park,
where British Canoeing and the National
Watersports Centre are based. The route goes
through the heart of the city and countryside,
passing some of Nottingham's most well-
known landmarks including Nottingham Castle,
Notts County and Nottingham Forest football
stadiums and the Boots HQ. There are three

locks: Meadow Lane, Castle and Beeston,
as well as a weir to portage. British Canoeing
launched the trail in 2016. As Adya reminds me,
Sian Sykes, founder of Psyched Paddleboarding
and one of the country's most well-respected
endurance paddleboarders, was the first to
take on the SUP challenge in October that year,
paddling clockwise to test her strength and
skills even further.

Adya and I have decided upon our shorter,
anticlockwise route, launching instead on to the
River Trent, the third longest river in the UK, by
County Hall at Victoria Embankment and close
to the beautiful, blue Trent Bridge. I've come
here by train from Yorkshire, taking a bus to the
famous Nottinghamshire County Cricket Club a
few minutes' walk away.

The river is busy with rowers, kayakers and
canoeists, and we are careful to paddle safely
along the right-hand side. About 200 metres
after the bridge we cross and leave the river
at the pontoon. We carry our boards through
the gate and make our way to the canal and
Meadow Lane Lock. I have a soft spot for urban
canals – the Birmingham canals are on my wish
list – and it feels like home as we paddle past
traditional narrowboats and under bridges,
seeing the industrial heritage of the city side by
side with new developments. Some may not like
the wall art; there are hard edges and at times
the distant roar of traffic; and we are unlikely to
spot a dolphin in the less-than-turquoise water.
But there is also beauty. One lesson the canals
have taught me is to look for the extraordinary
in the ordinary, to find the magic in mundane
places we might otherwise overlook. I take in
the yellow water lilies in the sunshine, three
ducks resting contentedly on a ledge and later
the stunning willow trees draping the towpath.

Opposite Adya under the Trent Bridge

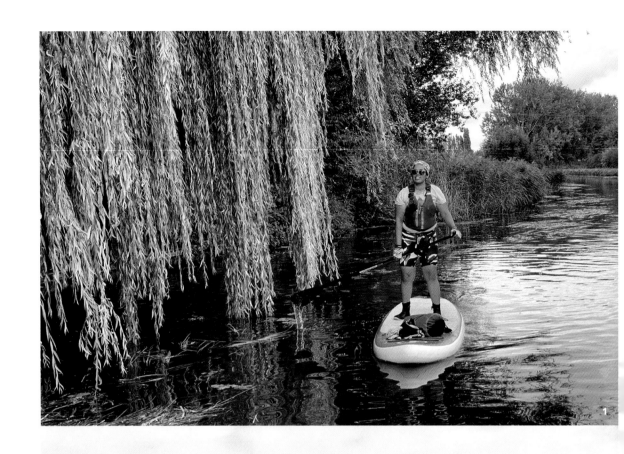

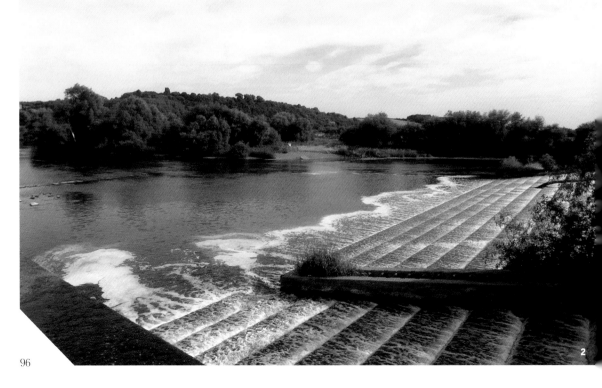

1 Paddling along the beautiful Nottingham and Beeston Canal   **2** Beeston Lock weir © Canalside Heritage Centre Trust

It's a joy to see the pretty, floating reed beds bringing colour and softness to the grey, concrete canal walls. Planted by Canal & River Trust volunteers and the Nottingham Narrowboat Project, they will attract bees and pollinating insects. The area was recently granted Green Flag Status by Keep Britain Tidy. They remind me of the award-winning work of the Wildlife Gardeners of Haggerston, creating gardens and habitats for birds, fish and insects at Kingsland Basin and Regent's Canal Nature Reserve in London.

There is a weekend buzz at the cafes on Castle Wharf as we pass the impressive Fellows, Morton & Clayton building. Once the largest canal transportation company in England, the warehouse became a canal museum before being converted to a real ale pub.

Portaging the Castle Lock and passing the Castle Marina, we reach a lovely stretch bustling with narrowboat owners enjoying the afternoon sunshine. Adya and I share the easy companionship of a long paddle, chatting side by side about her role as a British Canoeing #ShePaddles Club Champion, the water skills she brings to SUP from kayaking and the psychology behind being a coach. I graze happily, picking the ripe blackberries growing along the side of the canal.

We are soon at Beeston Lock where we stop for an ice cream in the sun close to the Attenborough Nature Reserve. I'd hoped to treat Adya to a late lunch at the Canalside Heritage Centre, an arts and education hub housed in the historic weir cottages, or the Boathouse Cafe at the marina, but we arrive a little too late. Something for another day.

It's now time to move from Nottingham and Beeston Canal to the River Trent at the weir, and as the water thunders behind us the river widens and we pass Clifton Hall on a hill on the right. The view before us is breathtaking. Lined with trees, the River Trent feels a world away from the city. We spot the bright blue of a kingfisher, watch herons perched on a low branch and see swans resting elegantly in the reeds. There is the odd plop of a fish jumping behind us.

'Come ride the water train!' calls Adya and together we find the strongest flow and fly along the river, realising that we go faster if we don't paddle. While a canal demands effort with every kilometre, the river rewards us with a little help. With a cheery hello to anglers along the side, we enjoy the peace and quiet, watching the clouds reflected in the river.

An hour later we are close to the busy Victoria Embankment and our launch (and now exit) point once more, with 17 kilometres of paddleboarding completed. My train leaves soon so we speedily pack up the boards and Adya kindly drops me back at the station. I run to the platform and throw myself and my board rather inelegantly into the carriage with a minute to spare before the doors close.

I'm grateful for the chance to snooze on the train after a longish day of paddling. The Trent Loop Challenge is one I would definitely recommend for its variety, history, beauty and sense of community. My only regret is not getting to Beeston Lock earlier to treat Adya – but then that leaves something to enjoy next time. Perhaps we'll see you there.

Technical information

DISTANCE **17km round trip.**

LAUNCH LOCATION
ENTRY AND EXIT POINT **SK 581381/52.938, -1.136**
TURN AROUND POINT **SK 536353/52.912, -1.204**

ALTERNATIVE ROUTE **You could break the route into different sections. Paddle part of the canal or river and be picked up, or ring for a taxi, at one of the locks. Alternatively, do a shuttle and leave one car at the exit point if there are two or more of you with cars.**

Difficulty

To complete the loop we paddled is physically demanding; paddleboarding on the river section especially takes planning, thought and an understanding of the obstacles and equipment required.

Getting there

Nottingham is widely connected by rail, bus and car. We launched from just in front of County Hall by Trent Bridge. This is about 2.5km from Nottingham railway station if you wish to walk. Buses from the railway station to Nottinghamshire Cricket Club stop at Bridgford Road and Radcliffe Road. If you are happy to carry your board, perhaps use the tram park and ride to Trent Bridge.

There is paid road parking on the Victoria Embankment (SK 573379/52.935, -1.148). For a fee you can park at the National Water Sports Centre (SK 611386/52.941, -1.091) – use the car park near the cafe and family fun park, following signs for the white water course. There is a slipway down to the river.

Route information

A Waterways Licence is required to paddle on the Nottingham and Beeston Canal and the River Trent.

British Canoeing's official Trent Loop Challenge is 20km.

To launch beneath Beeston Lock weir, walk down the path by the side of the Canalside Heritage Centre. Go to the middle of the river once launched as it is a little shallow by the edges, and keep a safe distance from the weir itself. There are public toilets a short distance from the lock.

Exiting the river at the pontoon by Trent Bridge isn't difficult, it is just a little awkward getting through the gate at the top.

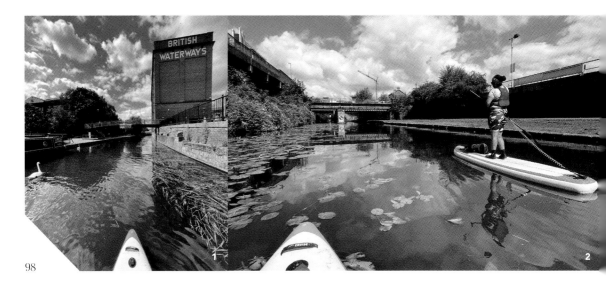

1 Scenic paddling through Nottingham   2 Water lilies on the Nottingham and Beeston Canal   3 Glassy water

Although the Nottingham and Beeston Canal and River Trent are in the same catchment, do inspect your boards as you move from the canal to the river for any plants and small insects. See British Canoeing information on the Check, Clean, Dry procedure and how to combat invasive species.

On canals keep to the right and be aware of boats in front and from behind. Pass port to port (left-hand side to left-hand side) with oncoming boats.

Eating and drinking
» The Boathouse Cafe at Beeston Marina comes highly recommended.
» Canalside Heritage Centre has a cafe, a beautiful garden and a shop, and runs events, such as honey extraction demonstrations, archaeology walks and bike maintenance.

Instruction, guided tours and equipment hire
» There are no paddleboard hire companies near where we launched. However, Adya is a SUP coach, blogger and YouTube kit reviewer at Just One More Paddle.

» For lessons and tours in the Nottingham area, check out Emma Love at WotBikini Stand Up Paddleboarding or SUP With Charlotte.
» You can also hire boards to use at the Holme Pierrepont Country Park lagoon or pay a fee to use your own board there.

Further information
» Sian Sykes, Psyched Paddleboarding: *www.psychedpaddleboarding.com*
» British Canoeing's Trent Loop Challenge: *www.gopaddling.info/ gopaddlingchallenges/trent-loop-challenge-route*
» Stand Up Paddle UK community: *www.instagram.com/standuppaddleuk*
» Wildlife Gardeners of Haggerston: *www.wildlifegardenersofhaggerston.org*
» Attenborough Nature Reserve: *www.nottinghamshirewildlife.org*

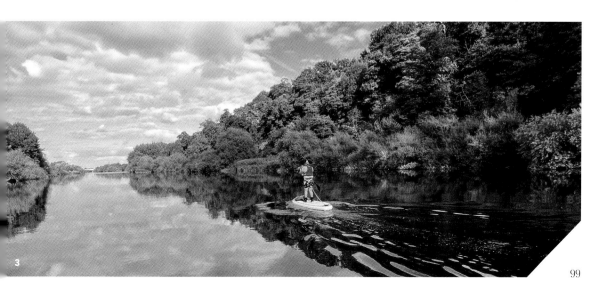

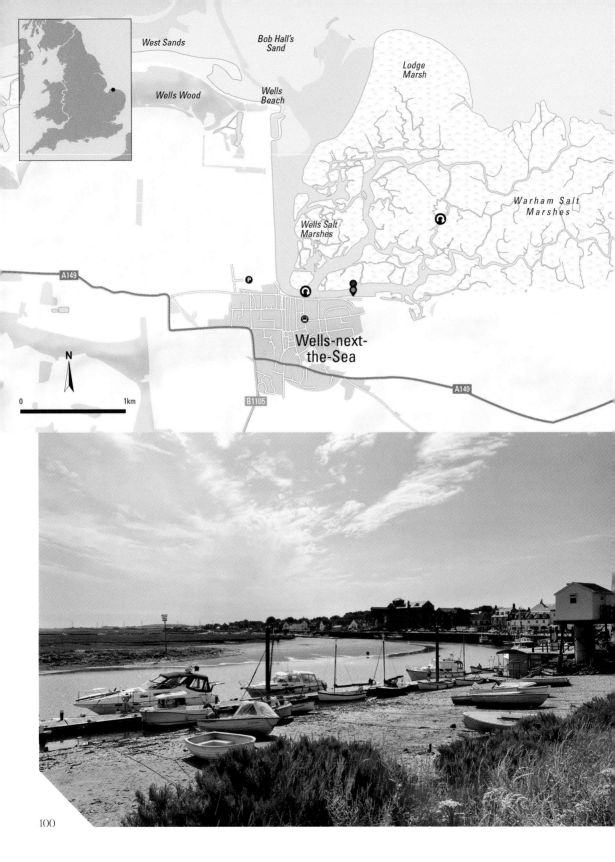

West Sands

Bob Hall's
Sand

Lodge
Marsh

Wells Wood

Wells
Beach

*Warham Salt
Marshes*

*Wells Salt
Marshes*

A149

Wells-next-
the-Sea

N

0   1km

A149

B1105

Wells-next-the-Sea

THE LIFEBOAT HORSE SCULPTURE, WHOOSHING THROUGH THE SALT MARSHES, SEA LAVENDER AND BEAUTIFUL BEACH HUTS

Bright-blue skies and sunshine greet me as I arrive at the quay in Wells-next-the-Sea, eager to meet Sam Rutt, highly accomplished SUP racer, founder of Barefoot SUP and Fitness and the first woman to paddleboard the Wash. I've come to paddle with her through the tidal salt marsh creeks and fishing harbour of this beautiful town on the north Norfolk coast.

Walking past families crabbing (or gillying), I look over to the sandbank and see the sculpture that has also drawn me here: Rachael Long's Lifeboat Horse. The three-metre-high horse was commissioned for the Wells Heritage Art Trail in 2018 and is made from steel bars and whisky barrels as a tribute to the historic lifeboat horses of the town. Discussing the brief for the trail, Harbour Master Robert Smith MBE (who I'm lucky enough to meet later) showed Rachael a photograph of five pairs of heavy horses pulling the Wells lifeboat. In the 1800s, rockets were fired to alert the lifeboat crew of a vessel in distress and the horses would gallop to the gate, ready to be led to the lifeboat house on the quay. From there they would pull the lifeboat the four kilometres to Holkham Gap where it could be launched. In 2019 the Wells community fundraised the £15,000 required to buy the horse and install it permanently on the sandbank. Donations came from businesses, local residents and even schoolchildren donating their pocket money, because, according to Robert Smith, 'so many people loved it'.

As the tide is out, I can see the sculpture standing proudly on the sand. In a few hours it will be partially submerged by the sea, looking as if it is moving through the waves. I have been looking forward to paddling close to it for so long.

I meet Sam at the east end of the quay, a short walk from John's Rock Shop and French's Fish and Chips. Sam is working with the Wells Harbour Commissioners to offer paddleboarding opportunities to young people in the community alongside building her business. As Wells is tidal, she also offers Zoom SUP safety events for paddleboarders, the proceeds of the ticket sales going to the RNLI. She introduces me to Robert Smith and we chat about his book *Crossing the Bar – Tales of Wells Harbour*.

The morning's gentle breeze has now picked up and Sam takes time to explain the impact of the wind, the tide, the boats and buoys we will paddle around and the channels on either side of the sandbank. We launch at the public slip by the Wells Harbour Commissioners an hour before high tide. This is one of two public slips you can launch from; the Wells Sailing Club slip, however, is for members only. We turn right and paddle towards the creeks. It feels like quite an adventure into a stunning landscape.

The north Norfolk coast is a designated Area of Outstanding Natural Beauty, and Wells sits within the 3,706 hectares of the Holkham National Nature Reserve. Pretty, purple sea lavender is in abundance, carpeting the marsh with its beauty. There is also bright-green samphire growing on the water's edge. In the distance we see the distinctive red sails of a Coastal Exploration Company boat, winding its way through the creeks. As we pass the Wells Ferry we say a cheery hello to the clients on board. The route twists and turns, and looking

Opposite Wells Harbour

back we have a wonderful view of the town. There is a warm breeze, blue sky and sunshine – it feels like a perfect summer's day exploring and chatting.

After about an hour it is time to change direction and head for the harbour. The energy we put into paddling into the wind will now be rewarded. As we return to the town, the wind is behind our backs and we soon feel like we are flying. My confidence has improved with my SUP fitness since Llyn Tegid (p23) and I follow Sam, giggling with excitement as we whoosh across the water.

We pass the slip where we launched and head to the Lifeboat Horse. The waves are lapping against its legs as it stands majestically on the sand. I feel quite moved to be able

to paddle so close and reflect upon the part horses have played in making Wells a safe haven. In the background we can see the retired lifeboats, which adds to the sense of history.

It is time to get back to the launch point and there is one final paddle into the wind as we return to the slip. Sam generously gives all her clients a small box of two Fortnum and Mason chocolates and I'm looking forward to savouring them back on dry land.

Having explored the creeks and harbour, I wander through the town to learn more and visit the wonderful arts, heritage and community centre Wells Maltings on Staithe Street. I take a few moments to walk through the interesting exhibition about the town's history, geography and famous faces. With a

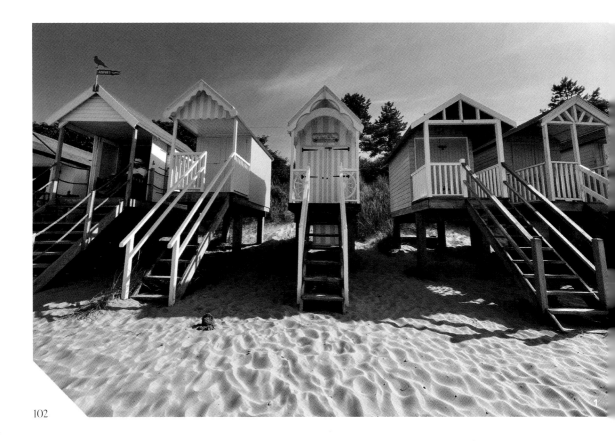

1 Pretty beach huts   **2** A sunny day at Wells Harbour

cafe and small shop, it is a lovely spot for a cup of tea and cake or lunch.

The creeks and Lifeboat Horse have drawn me to Wells, but there is one more place I am keen to walk to: the award-winning beach. A kilometre and a half from the town, it is known for its beautiful pine forest, dunes and brightly coloured beach huts. I am not sure I have ever walked in sand that feels so soft. A new boathouse is being built by the beach which will house Wells's new Shannon-class lifeboat, to be called the *Duke of Edinburgh* in memory of Prince Philip's commitment to maritime services. The names of 10,000 loved ones will also be displayed on the boat's hull as part of the RNLI's fundraising Launch a Memory campaign.

As I make my way back to the quay, I notice a woman sitting on the grass looking out to sea. 'I hope you don't mind me telling you this,' I say, 'but you look the picture of peace and happiness.'

'Thank you,' she replies, smiling. 'I live by the sea but am visiting friends here in Wells. Peace and happiness are exactly how I feel every time I come here.'

I can understand why she feels like this. Paddleboarding through the salt marshes and sea lavender, walking on the beach and seeing the Lifeboat Horse have been a joy – a safe haven indeed. I hope you'll treat yourself to a day in Wells and will feel that same peace and happiness too.

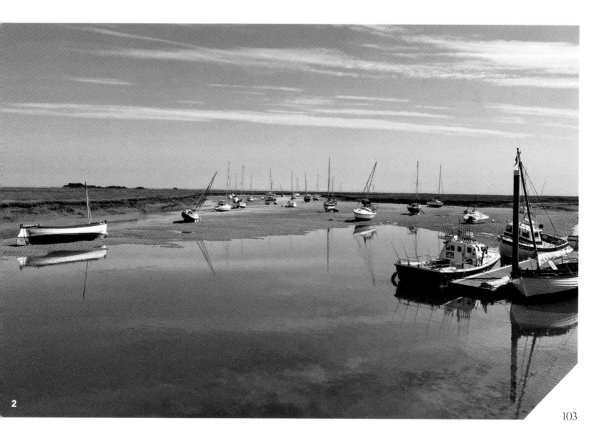

2

Technical information

DISTANCE **5.5km round trip.**

LAUNCH LOCATION:
ENTRY AND EXIT POINT **TF 923438/52.957, 0.862**
TURN AROUND POINT 1 **TF 931445/52.963, 0.874**
TURN AROUND POINT 2 **TF 918438/52.957, 0.853**

Difficulty

Paddleboarding experience is necessary for this trip and knowledge of wind and tides is important for Wells salt marshes if going independently. Be careful to use the salt marsh channels so as not to damage them. The Harbour Office sells tide timetables for Wells.

Getting there

The nearest railway stations are Sheringham and King's Lynn, with connections to Norwich and London respectively. Buses throughout Norfolk, including buses to King's Lynn and Fakenham, stop 650m away on Standard Road.

There is a pay-and-display car park on Wells's quay, owned by the Port of Wells and operated by a private contractor (TF 913439/52.959, 0.846).

Route information

There are RNLI lifeguards at Wells Beach but not in the harbour.

Wells Harbour Commissioners has a webcam.

Eating and drinking

» The Wells Maltings houses a lovely cafe serving breakfast, lunch and cakes.

Instruction, guided tours and equipment hire

» Sam Rutt at Barefoot SUP and Fitness offers SUP beginners and progression courses, guided tours in Wells and SUP fitness and race training courses, as well as SUP safety online Zoom events.
» North Norfolk Paddle Boards runs lessons and guided tours from Burnham Overy Staithe, Stiffkey and Brancaster, including breakfast and sunset SUP sessions.
» Norfolk Outdoor Adventures, based on the Norfolk Broads, offers SUP beginners and skills and progression classes, sunset SUP adventures and an introduction to coastal SUP workshop. It only hires boards to clients who have been on its classes.
» Norfolk Paddle Boards, based in Norwich, offers lessons, sunset SUP tours and SUP socials as well as board hire.

Further information

» Rachael Long:
  www.rachaellongsculpture.com
» Coastal Exploration Company:
  www.coastalexplorationcompany.co.uk
» Wells Harbour Tours:
  www.wellsharbourtours.com
» Robert Smith MBE, *Crossing the Bar – Tales of Wells Harbour* (self-published, 2018).

Opposite Sam paddleboarding just by Wells

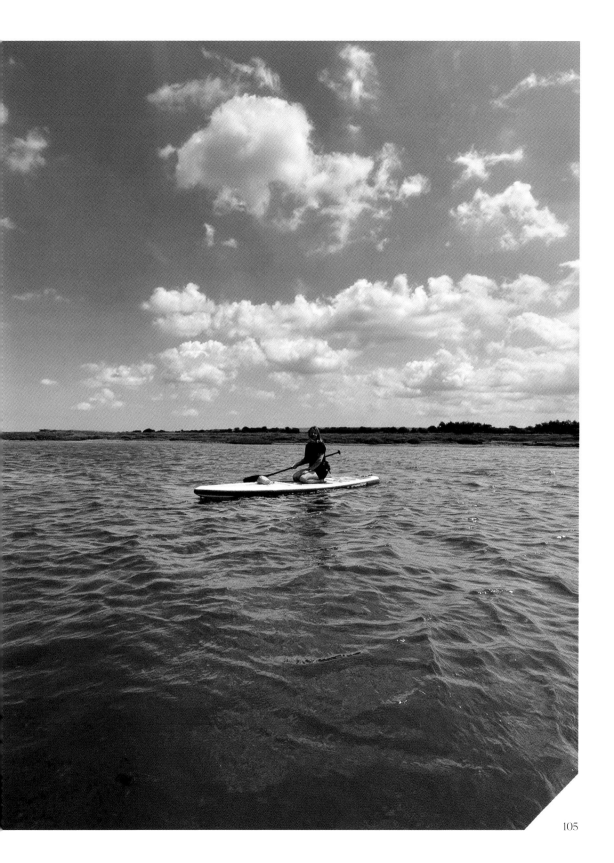

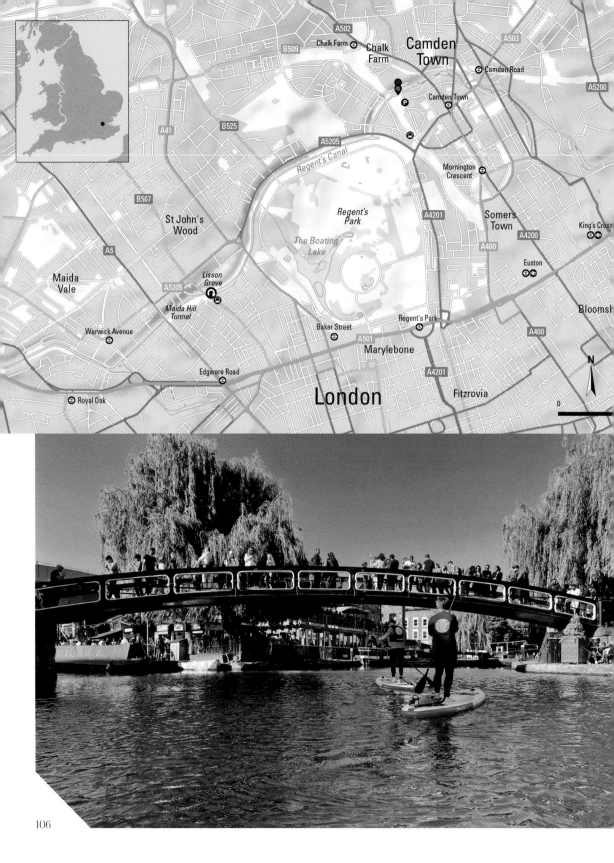

Regent's Canal, London

**URBAN SUP ADVENTURES, THE PIRATE CASTLE,
COMMUNITY AND CONNECTION ON THE CANAL
AND LOOKING OUT FOR THE GIRAFFES**

It's a sunny, late-Sunday afternoon and I've come to England's capital to paddleboard along Regent's Canal with Anu, Josh and the social SUP club from Paddleboarding London. We pass the 'guitar guy' on The Music Boat, singing his enthusiastic rendition of 'London's Calling' by The Clash. His passengers on the punt wave and smile at us. The towpath is buzzing with London life. It feels like we are both a part of and apart from it in our peaceful world on the water.

At just under 14 kilometres, Regent's Canal runs through London from Little Venice to the Docklands. Completed in 1820, it is named after the Prince Regent (later George IV) and links the Paddington Arm of the Grand Union Canal, which starts in Birmingham some 220 kilometres away, with the River Thames in London. From its pretty collection of narrowboats moored at Little Venice's Blomfield Road, the canal passes the edge of Regent's Park and ZSL London Zoo. A huge aviary is being refurbished on one side and on the other you are invited to look out for the hunting dogs – friends have even spotted the odd giraffe. According to an ecologist I speak to the next day, the bushes along the canal are home to the non-native Aesculapian snake, found only in two other places in the UK.

Further on in Camden, famous for its market, cafes and eclectic shops, the canal then runs to the redeveloped King's Cross. Here you can enjoy the wonderful Word on the Water floating bookshop, a 1920s Dutch barge filled with books, a friendly parrot and cosy stove. From there the canal drops down to meet the River Thames at Limehouse.

Paddleboarding London is based at the Pirate Castle, a 500-metre walk from Camden Town tube station. It is the home of the Pirate Castle charity that is committed to making the waterways available to more people, with a focus on children, young people and SEND (special educational needs and disability) groups of all ages. Every time a board is booked, Paddleboarding London donates to their work.

We launch from the pontoon at the castle. Designed by the famous architect Richard Seifert and constructed in 1977, it has been referred to as the first defensive castle to be built since the sixteenth century. We head west towards Maida Hill Tunnel, passing the beautiful houses and gardens of Primrose Hill, some of which have their own moorings. The walls and bridges along the canal have some spectacular street art and we can hear the echo of pigeons cooing on the steelwork. This is urban exploring on a SUP. As we paddle along, Anu, co-owner of Paddleboarding London, tells me how city waterways offer a chance to find joy, well-being and adventure on our doorstep in the city, even better as they can be reached without a car.

At the Feng Shang Princess, a floating, three-tier pagoda at Cumberland Basin, we bear right. At this point the Cumberland Arm of the canal used to lead to Cumberland Market, London's primary hay and straw market, in the 1800s. The market went into decline and in 1938 the canal was dammed off and drained. Rubble from the London Blitz was used to fill it and this was later covered in topsoil from Windsor Castle as the area was turned into allotments.

Ahead lies a stretch of canal lined with beautiful willow trees, the branches gently touching the ripples on the water as we pass

Opposite A beautiful day of SUP in the city

through ZSL London Zoo. The towpath is busy with walkers, cyclists and runners: families and friends stroll along chatting in the sunshine; a couple picnicking on a bench hold hands. The blue and green ribbon of the canal is bringing people together in the heart of the capital.

The waterways have their own community and Anu guides and advises us on the boat traffic. As paddleboarders we paddle down the middle of the canal, moving to the right when a boat passes. There are the waterbuses as well as the canal touring boats *Jason's Trip* and *Jenny Wren* carrying passengers along the canal and GoBoats which can be hired for private parties. The speed limit is six kilometres per hour, which shouldn't create a wash, but it is always better to keep a keen eye out for boats that may not see you. Anu knows people on and off the water too, chatting to an angler we pass and locals sunbathing on the towpath.

We soon arrive at Lisson Grove, a Canal & River Trust gated mooring for the community living side by side on their narrowboats. Flowers and plants blossom by the boats and it feels a huge privilege to paddle past their homes. At the gates of the grove lie old bikes, motorbikes and the odd trolley lifted from the canal by magnet fishing. A fascinating collection – I wonder what stories they could tell.

Pre-authorisation is required to SUP through the 249-metre Maida Hill Tunnel, so we turn back to Camden. You could of course portage your board to Little Venice and paddle on to Paddington. On our right, six magnificent, Quinlan Terry-designed villas stand tall on their manicured gardens. We pass back under the Macclesfield Bridge, known as Blow Up Bridge – at 3 a.m. on 2 October 1874, a barge called *Tilbury* carrying coffee, nuts, petroleum and gunpowder set alight, resulting in the deaths

of three men on board. The bridge was rebuilt with the original pillars, but with one significant difference: the pillars were turned around to offer a smooth side for the ropes used to tow boats, so you'll now see grooves on both sides.

'Shall we go to Camden?' Anu suggests, and of course we are all keen. We paddle on near the old gin distillery founded by Walter and Alfred Gilbey in 1857, which has been redeveloped into homes. She also points out the entrance to a tunnel, part of the Camden Catacombs, an underground network of passageways and engine vaults that allowed horses to move safely and work at Euston railway station. As we return to the Pirate Castle, there's music, dancing and laughter on the towpath. We say our goodbyes and wish each other well for the week ahead.

The next morning I return to Camden to walk along the canal through Little Venice and Paddington. Enjoying a cup of tea at the cafe in the beautiful gardens of St Mark's Church, I reflect upon what Anu had said. Paddleboarding along Regent's Canal isn't the aspirational turquoise waters and ocean views many associate with SUP. What it offers instead is a sense of community, history, beauty and calm right in the heart of London. Feeling connected to others and to place is such an important part of the human experience and paddleboarding in the capital with Anu and her social SUP club I felt that. This is blue health in the city. Next time I'm in London I'll book a SUP yoga lesson in St Katharine Docks or a moonlight paddle with Anu. I'd love to explore more of the canal from Little Venice to Paddington and King's Cross. If London's calling, my answer will always be a definite 'yes'. I hope it will be for you too.

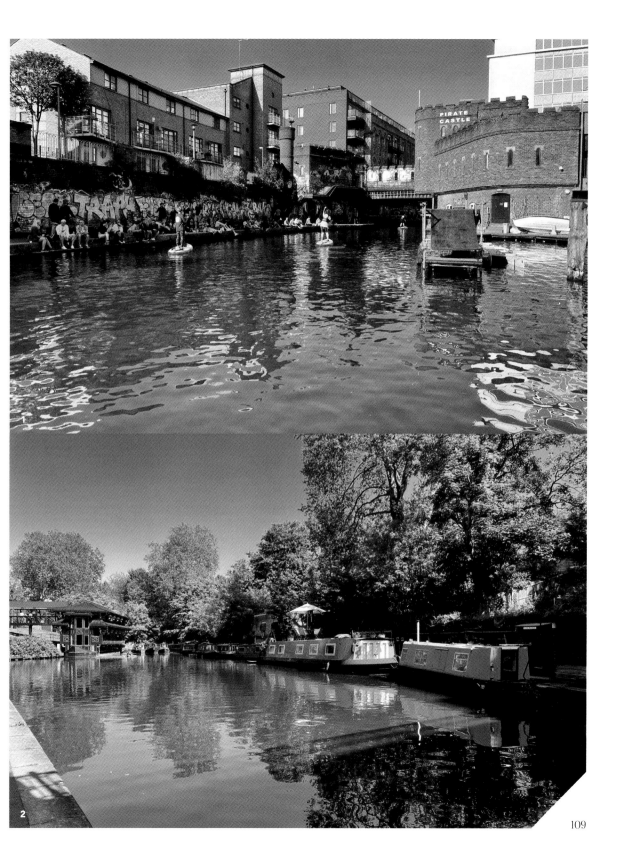

Technical information

DISTANCE **4.75km round trip.**

LAUNCH LOCATION
ENTRY AND EXIT POINT **TQ 285840/51.540, -0.148**
TURN AROUND POINT **TQ 270824/51.526, -0.171**

Difficulty
This is a lovely paddle for beginners and more experienced paddleboarders alike wanting to explore the capital's canals. Be aware of boats and anglers.

Getting there
Camden can be reached by tube and bus as well as by car. The nearest tube station to the Pirate Castle is Camden Town. There are bike racks on Oval Road and bike sharing stations nearby.

There is parking available around the Pirate Castle for two hours maximum (TQ 285839/51.540, -0.1481).

Route information
Please note that launching from the pontoon at the Pirate Castle is only available to customers of Paddleboarding London. If you wish to SUP here independently there are plenty of places to launch from the towpath and I met a couple of paddleboarders who regularly do this – simply walk down the steps from Oval Road. To give yourself space to pump up your board I would advise getting there early in the day, as the towpath does get busy. You will need a Waterways Licence.

Eating and drinking
» Camden has lots of great cafes. I had a delicious lunch at It's All Greek to Me! in the North Yard.
» St Mark's Church garden cafe can be reached from the canal towpath or Prince Albert Road.

Instruction, guided tours and equipment hire
» Paddleboarding London offers SUP lessons, tours and SUP yoga. It does not hire boards but does hold supervised SUP sessions.
» Active360 at Merchant Square in nearby Paddington Basin offers lessons and board hire for experienced paddleboarders. It works out of Kew Bridge and Brentford Lock as well, where it offers lessons, tours and board hire. If you want to paddle on the River Thames, Active360 offers Thames skills and knowledge courses.

Further information
» The Pirate Castle: *www.thepiratecastle.org*
» The Music Boat: *www.themusicboat.org*
» Word on the Water: *www.wordonthewater.co.uk*
» Canal & River Trust: *www.canalrivertrust.org.uk*

Opposite Macclesfield Bridge

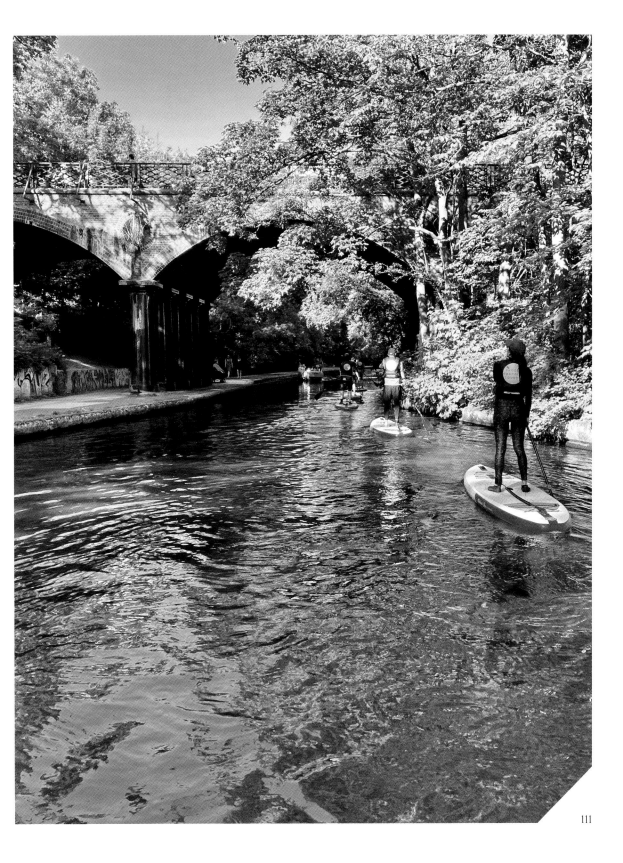

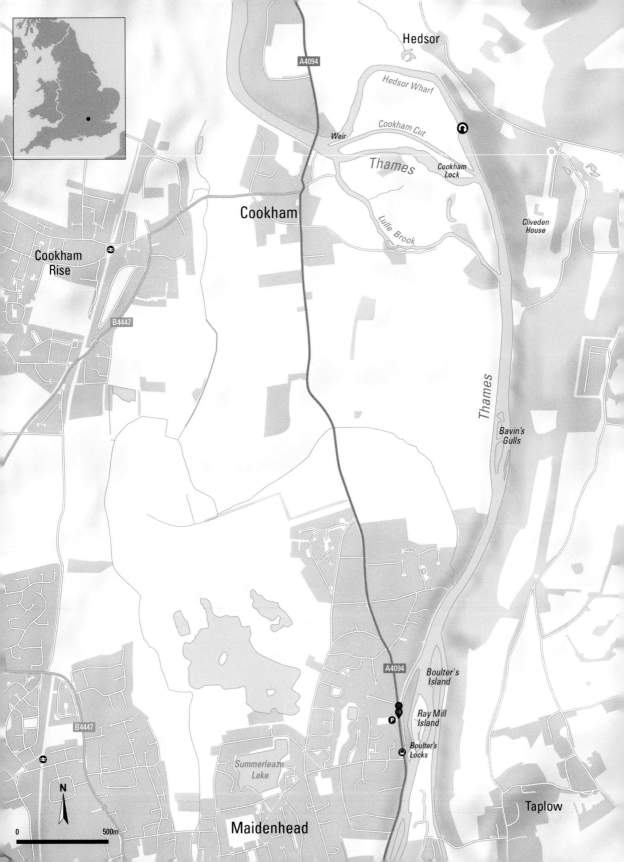

Hedsor

A4094

Hedsor Wharf

Cookham Cut

Weir

Thames

Cookham Lock

Cookham

Lulle Brook

Cliveden House

Cookham Rise

B4447

Thames

Bavin's Gulls

Boulter's Island

A4094

Ray Mill Island

P

Summerleaze Lake

Boulter's Locks

N

Taplow

0   500m

Maidenhead

Maidenhead and Cliveden House, River Thames

CLIVEDEN HOUSE, A BLUE COTTAGE WITH ROSES AROUND THE DOOR, 'GUARDIANS OF THE THAMES' AND PADDLEBOARDING 'THE SWEETEST STRETCH OF ALL THE RIVER'

'Don't you just feel the problems of the world float away the minute you get on your paddleboard?' says Cath as we launch on to the River Thames. Given she has recently completed a demanding fundraising SUP adventure down the River Wye with her school friend Ginny Cooper, it's lovely to hear that paddleboarding still holds the same magic for her.

'I do,' I reply, 'absolutely.'

I've come to Maidenhead to paddle with Cath Knight, mum of two teenage sons, from Boulter's Lock to Hedsor Wharf, passing Cliveden House and the National Trust estate that surrounds it. Ahead of our day together, Cath sends me a quote from Jerome K Jerome's book *Three Men in a Boat* in which he describes the route: 'in its unbroken loveliness this is, perhaps, the sweetest stretch of all the river'.

Our mutual friend Martin Dorey, founder of the 2 Minute Foundation, messages me after paddling the same route with Cath with a simple, 'It's fab!' I head south from Yorkshire with growing excitement.

The River Thames is the longest river wholly in England and the second longest in Britain after the River Severn. Measuring 346 kilometres, its source is Trewsbury Mead in the Cotswold Hills. From there it flows through Oxford, Reading, Henley-on-Thames, Windsor and London and then joins the North Sea via the Thames Estuary. It has over 200 bridges, two foot tunnels at Greenwich and Woolwich and 45 locks on the non-tidal stretch, 40 of

which have resident lock-keepers. There are around 180 islands, also called eyots or aits, and our journey will start from one of them, Boulter's Island, which was once home to the broadcaster Richard Dimbleby. From Teddington Lock in west London, the river becomes tidal and is known as the Tideway or tidal Thames. With two tides a day, the water levels rise and fall by as much as seven metres.

In 2015, friends Michelle Ellison and Melanie Joe paddleboarded the entire length of the River Thames from its source to Southend-on-Sea, after the Port of London Authority had placed a ban on stand-up paddleboarding through central London in 2010. They tested the quality of the water along the way, reporting their findings to Thames21, a charity committed to cleaning the 644-kilometre network of London's waterways which works with approximately 7,000 volunteers every year.

I asked Michelle to tell me more about the challenge: 'We were determined to show that the River Thames could be paddleboarded safely from source to sea and worked for months with the Port of London Authority to research and plan for new safety measures, allowing us and those following to SUP the length of this most epic and beautiful river. It is rich with wildlife, friendly lock-keepers, boat owners and ramblers along the towpath. Plus, of course, there are the delicious riverside pubs like that at Boulter's Lock.'

It is at Boulter's Lock that Cath and I begin our own Thames adventure, launching opposite the car park near Dimbleby's old home, where a plaque marks the spot. A charming statue of a chap relaxing on a garden chair greets us.

1 Spring Cottage on the Cliveden estate © @supcoach_belle   **2** The lush River Thames

We head upstream towards Cliveden House, leaving the busyness of the world behind us.

It is a slightly overcast Thursday morning and the river feels peaceful. We paddle along chatting about Cath's River Wye challenge fundraising for Live Kindly Live Loudly in memory of Ruby Fuller, a young woman who died of leukemia aged 18. She tells me it has made her feel braver and more determined to embrace life to the full. The river is lined with beech, sycamore and willow trees; there are yellow water lilies growing along the edge and in the clear water I see the reeds swaying in the gentle flow. Every so often there is the familiar plop of a fish behind us. Geese line up along the bank preening themselves and swans glide past nonchalantly.

In a couple of weeks, the annual Swan Upping will take place. Travelling in traditional rowing skiffs and wearing the scarlet uniform of the Queen, the Queen's Swan Marker David Barber and his team will spend five days collecting data on the swans, assessing the health of the cygnets, treating the injured and teaching local primary schools about conservation of the river.

As we gently paddle along, the majesty of Cliveden House comes into view ahead, standing proudly above Cliveden Woods. It is breathtaking and it feels special to have such a spectacular vantage point from our boards. The 376 acres of the Cliveden House estate were gifted to the National Trust in 1942 by William Waldorf Astor and are open to visitors. Some of their Canadian canoes, rowing boats and electric boats are being rented, and they join us on the water.

We paddle to the right and wind our way

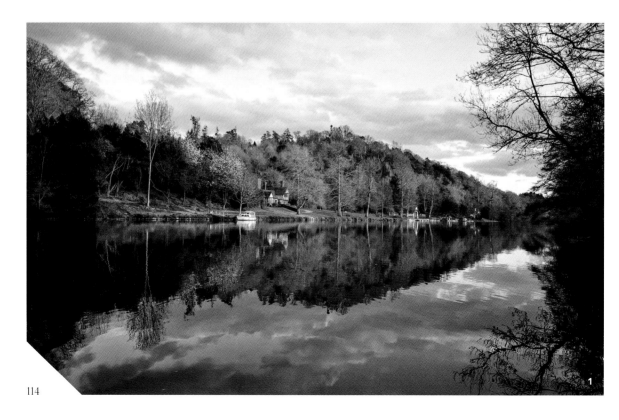

1

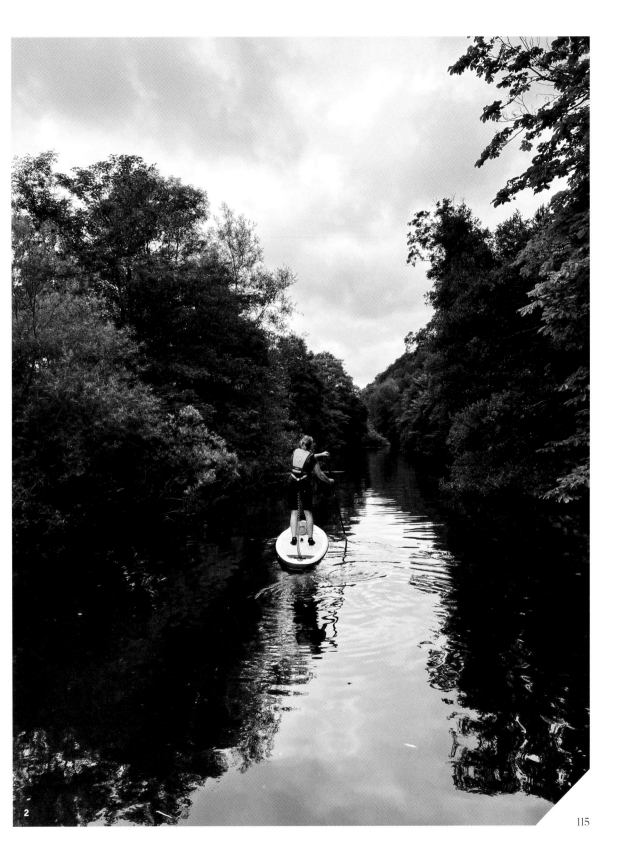

1 Perfect paddling conditions © @supcoach_belle   **2** Approaching Hedsor Wharf

through the four narrow islands at Bavin's Gulls, also known as Sloe Grove Islands, where a boat is moored, its washing drying on the line. As we approach Hedsor Wharf, Cath tells me to look out for the cottages on the riverbank. A simple brown building is followed by an immaculate blue cottage with roses around the door and a pretty rowing boat moored in front. If Little Bo-Peep had stepped out of the porch, it would not have surprised me. We take a moment to soak up the beauty and enjoy one of Cath's homemade bliss balls, then turn back to Boulter's Lock. A few more people are now enjoying the river: paddleboarders, a couple of cruisers, a rowing boat and narrowboat. On a sunny summer's weekend, I imagine this stretch could get very busy and we would need to watch out for the traffic and its wake. For now, though, we paddle along peacefully, inspecting the narrowboat for sale by the towpath and wondering what it might be like to live permanently on the river.

As we deflate my board before going for lunch at the Lake House Cafe at nearby Taplow Lake, we meet Tara Crist, founder of Paddleboard Maidenhead. Her business runs SUP courses, guided tours and SUP yoga retreats along the River Thames. She tells us about an educational paddleboarding day she is about to hold for a local school, teaching students about the history, geology and ecology of the river, how it has shaped the lives of generations of people living nearby and how they as 'guardians of the Thames' can make a difference to its future. A paddleboarding history and conservation lesson sounds so much more appealing than the PE lessons I had in the 1970s and 1980s.

A few weeks later Cath shares the news that she has qualified as a SUP instructor and is now taking beginners along the stretch we paddled together. I ring to congratulate her and recall how she said her adventure on the River Wye for Ruby's Live Kindly Live Loudly legacy had encouraged her to embrace life's opportunities. Maybe SUP has that effect. Maybe it helps us all live more fully and more bravely.

Who knows where paddleboarding on the River Thames may take you one day? From source to sea or to a new career. The stretch to Cliveden House would certainly be a beautiful place to start.

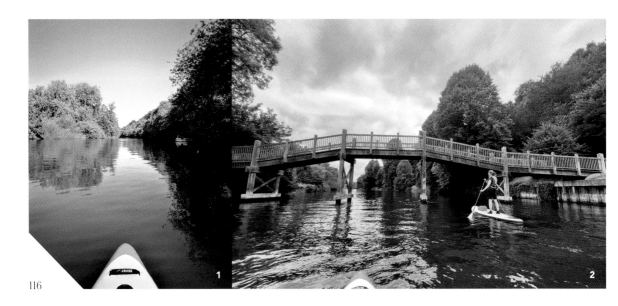

Technical information

DISTANCE **7km round trip.**

....

LAUNCH LOCATION
ENTRY AND EXIT POINT **SU 902825/51.535, -0.700**
TURN AROUND POINT **SU 906857/51.562, -0.694**

Difficulty

Paddleboarding on rivers takes planning and an understanding of the obstacles and the equipment required. Keep away from the weir close to the launch point. This route does not take you through any locks.

Getting there

The closest railway stations are Maidenhead or Taplow, with connections throughout London, just over 3km away. There is a frequent bus from Maidenhead railway station to Boulter's Lock.

You can reach Boulter's Lock by car along the Lower Cookham Road in Maidenhead. There is a pay-and-display car park, with a vehicle height restriction, right opposite the launch point at Boulter's Lock (SU 902825/51.535, -0.702). Be aware that Lower Cookham Road is very busy with traffic as you cross.

Route information

You will need a Waterways Licence. Port of London Authority require that all paddle-boarders wear a quick-release belt system rather than a calf or ankle leash on the tidal Thames

Eating and drinking

» We had a lovely lunch at the Lake House Cafe at Taplow Lake.
» The Boathouse at Boulter's Lock is a pub and restaurant good for food or just a drink.
» Ray Mill Island at the western bank of Boulter's Lock is lovely for ice cream and there are public toilets.

Instruction, guided tours and equipment hire

» Paddleboard Maidenhead runs beginner and improver classes, guided tours, SUP yoga retreats and safety, skills and rescue classes on the River Thames, as well as educational tours for young people.
» Gutsy Girls runs beginner lessons and hosts SUP socials along the River Thames at Richmond.
» Taplow Lakeside offers SUP hire.
» Active360, based at Kew Bridge, has created a Thames skill and knowledge course, developed with the Port of London Authority, to give you the knowledge to prepare to SUP on the tidal River Thames.

Further information

» Thames21: *www.thames21.org.uk*
» Live Kindly Live Loudly: *www.livekindlyliveloudly.co.uk*
» Thames Path: *www.nationaltrail.co.uk*
» Michelle and Mel have written an adventure blueprint of their source to Southend-on-Sea challenge: *www.shellsellison.com*
» Mark Rainsley, *Paddle the Thames: A guide for canoes, kayaks and SUPs* (Pesda Press, 2017).
» For more information on weather and river conditions, look at *www.paddleboardmaidenhead.uk* and the Environment Agency *riverconditions. environment-agency.gov.uk*

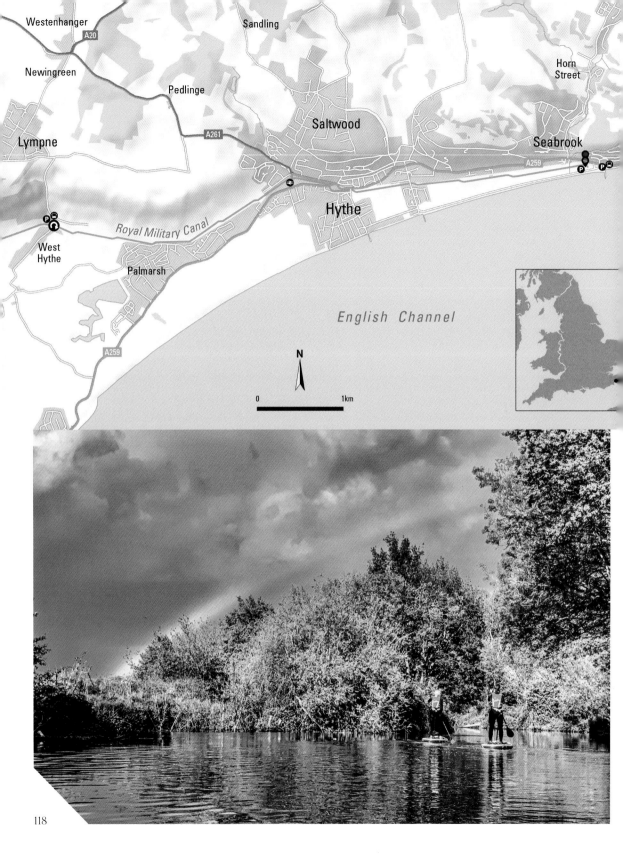

Royal Military Canal, Kent

SURPRISES IN THE GARDEN OF ENGLAND, SUP YOGA, A ZIGZAG CANAL AND A LITTER-PICKING PADDLETRIP

'Welcome to Hythe! On this side of the road we have the sea and this side the canal,' she says, smiling in the sunshine, her arms outstretched. 'Whatever the weather, we can paddleboard.'

It's a glorious day on the English south-east coast in Kent and I have come to meet presenter, podcast host and SUP yoga teacher India Pearson, who is going to share a very special place with me: the Royal Military Canal. On a summer's day in 2020, India paddleboarded the 45 kilometres of the canal, picking up and logging all the litter she found for the environmental charity Planet Patrol and fundraising for the 2 Minute Foundation.

It was the lush, green reeds and trees of the canal that India shared on her film *#LitterpickPaddletrip* that drew me to this part of Kent. I was also intrigued by the possibility of being able to paddleboard on both the sea and the canal in one day: they are quite literally divided by a beach, road and car park. If there is too much wind on the coast, the canal also offers a more sheltered paddleboarding experience. Two for one!

The Royal Military Canal was built between 1804 and 1809 as the third line of defence against the French in the Napoleonic Wars, the first being the Royal Navy patrolling the English Channel and the second the 74 Martello towers (small, defensive forts) built along the coast. It runs from Seabrook, near Folkestone in Kent, through Romney Marsh to Cliff End, near Hastings in East Sussex. 'Navigators', workmen who travelled the country building canals and railways at the time, dug the canal by hand, while the military built the ramparts. There

was also a towpath along its entire length for horses to pull the barges, which is now a lovely footpath for walkers. Interestingly, the canal has a unique shape as every 500 metres it bends, which allowed cannons to be fired with some protection; from the air it looks like a zigzag pattern. By the time it was completed, Britain was fighting in Spain and so it was never used as a military defence.

Today the Royal Military Canal is a haven for some of the beautiful wildlife of the Romney Marsh, the 260-square-kilometre wetland area in Kent and South East England. Part of the canal has been designated a Site of Special Scientific Interest and the rest a Local Wildlife Site. It is home to kingfishers, mute swans, marsh frogs and freshwater fish such as carp, pike, perch and eels.

After launching at the pontoon at the Seapoint Canoe Centre at the start of the canal, we paddle along under blue skies, saying hello to other paddleboarders and walkers. There is a gentle, countryside feel, with the grassy embankment sloping to the water on our right with areas set up for picnic tables and the towpath to our left. Beautiful pink water lilies line the side of the canal, damselflies and dragonflies dart among the reeds and there are swans and cygnets in the distance. If you are looking for a relaxing paddle, perhaps with friends or family walking along the towpath beside you, this is the perfect place. Whatever is going on in the world around you, this feels like an opportunity for calm and contemplation, a far cry from the reason the canal was originally built.

India, who has just told me the lovely news that she is pregnant, takes a moment to share some of her SUP yoga routine with me and

Opposite A surprise rainbow © @paddlecabin

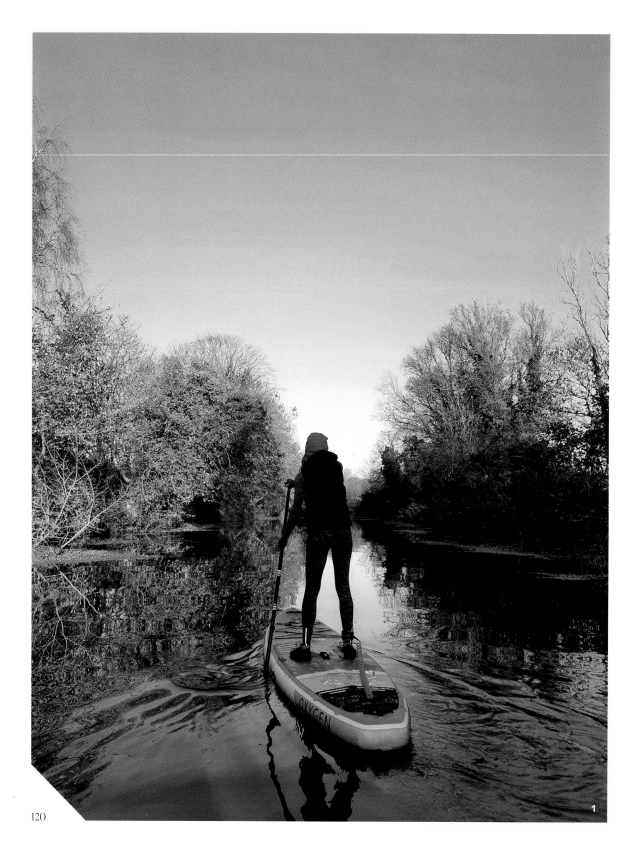

1 India on the beautiful canal © @with_india   **2** A gentle paddle on the Royal Military Canal

we chat about the benefits of yoga, Pilates and meditation on a paddleboard for our well-being. As we return to the launch point we meet a friend of hers who has been litter picking from the canal, inspired by India's challenge the year before.

It's time for lunch and we head to Unit 1, a brewery near West Hythe, where India had stopped to unload part of her plastic haul on her trip, including a pair of fishing waders and boots that were later upcycled to bags.

A SUP day out from our launch point to the cafe, paddling out and back or, like India, launching from the Hastings end and journeying to the cafe or along the length of the canal, are different options the canal offers. On more sheltered waterways like these, there are so many possibilities to start small and build up your skills and endurance.

We say our goodbyes as I go to explore the beach, picking up some bread for my picnics from Docker Bakery nearby. My next stop is further north in East Peckham and the River Medway.

Known as the 'Garden of England', inland Kent didn't immediately spring to mind when choosing places to research, which is why I find myself driving through an industrial estate the next day to visit the Paddle Cabin, a paddleboarding school on the banks of the River Medway. I'm curious to learn more. With a nearby cafe, it is bustling with SUP activity as members chat, pump boards and launch on to the river in the sunshine. Friends Jo and Hayley founded the business and offer tuition, coaching, club socials, SUP meditation and SUP yoga with India, as well as paddles to the pub, SUP pup sessions and tours along the river and further afield.

Jo also takes some time to kindly tell me about their favourite places to paddle in the county. They are two easily accessible places to launch along the River Medway: Tonbridge Lower Castle Field car park and Teston Bridge Country Park. Hayley is a huge fan of St Andrews Lakes, 70 acres of azure freshwater in Halling in the North Downs, where you can also swim, fish and even freedive or scuba dive.

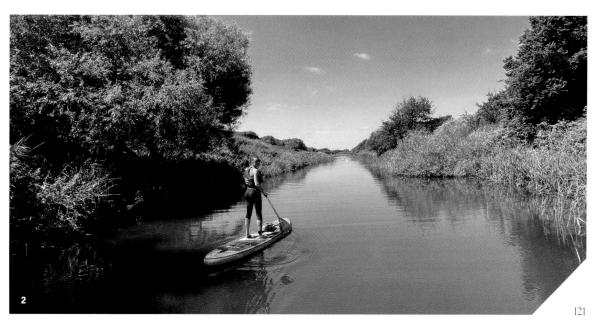

1 Paddleboarding joy © @with_india   **2** Water lilies   **3** All smiles on the Royal Military Canal

The lake used to be a quarry and the vibrant blue is thought to come from the limestone chalk in the cement-making process. They both love paddling through Canterbury along the River Stour, past the cathedral, under the city's bridges and then into the countryside, with a stop at a favourite pub along the way.

Once again, I am reminded how easy it is to overlook the magic of adventure and nature on our doorstep and how waterways created in different centuries, such as the Royal Military Canal, can offer paddleboarding and well-being possibilities today. It wasn't first on my list of places to research for you, but I am so glad I came to explore both coastal and inland Kent. Now to book a SUP yoga class ...

Technical Information

DISTANCE **13km round trip.**

LAUNCH LOCATION
ENTRY AND EXIT POINT **TR 188349/51.072, 1.122**
TURN AROUND POINT **TR 126342/51.068, 1.033**

Difficulty
The canal is a great spot for beginners and anyone looking to build up their skills and confidence.

Getting there
The closest railway stations to Hythe are Sandling and Folkestone West, both with connections to London. Buses to Hythe, Dover, Canterbury and Folkestone all stop a few hundred metres from the launch point.

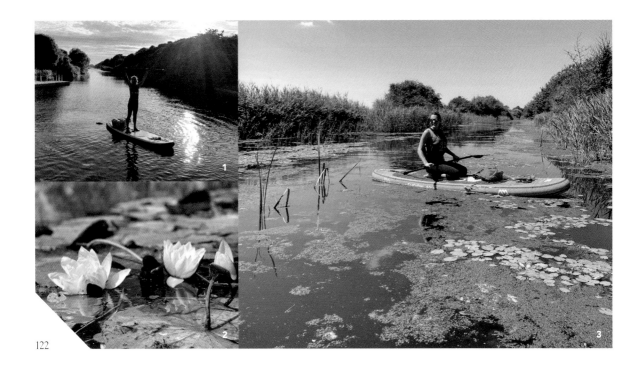

4 A sunny paddle

There is a pay-and-display car park called Sea Point car park by the canal on Princes Parade (TR 190349/51.071, 1.125).

There are public toilets along the esplanade towards the Hythe Imperial Hotel on Stade Street.

Route information

You must have a licence from Folkestone and Hythe District Council if you wish to use a paddleboard between Seabrook Outfall and West Hythe Dam on the Royal Military Canal. In 2022, this costs £19.50 for three months or £29.50 for a year. A British Canoeing membership will cover you from West Hythe Dam onwards towards Pett Level. However, India would not recommend paddling between Rye and Pett Level if you are not experienced as Rye is a tidal harbour and could be dangerous. Portage your board after West Hythe Dam.

Eating and drinking

» We had a lovely lunch at Unit 1, which sells drinks, cream teas and pizzas and has different pop-up cafes each weekend.
» Docker Bakery sells bread, flour, coffee and a delicious date, oat and chocolate slice.

Instruction, guided tours and equipment hire

» Seapoint Canoe Centre offers tuition and paddleboard hire.
» The SUP Hub offers tuition, guided tours on the sea and canal, paddleboard hire and community paddling.
» Paddle Cabin offers tuition, guided tours on the river, SUP events plus self-launch and board hire for members of the cabin community.

Further information

» Planet Patrol: *www.planetpatrol.co*
» 2 Minute Foundation: *www.beachclean.net*

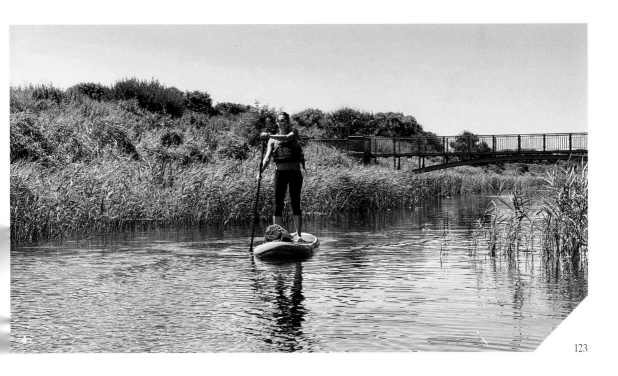

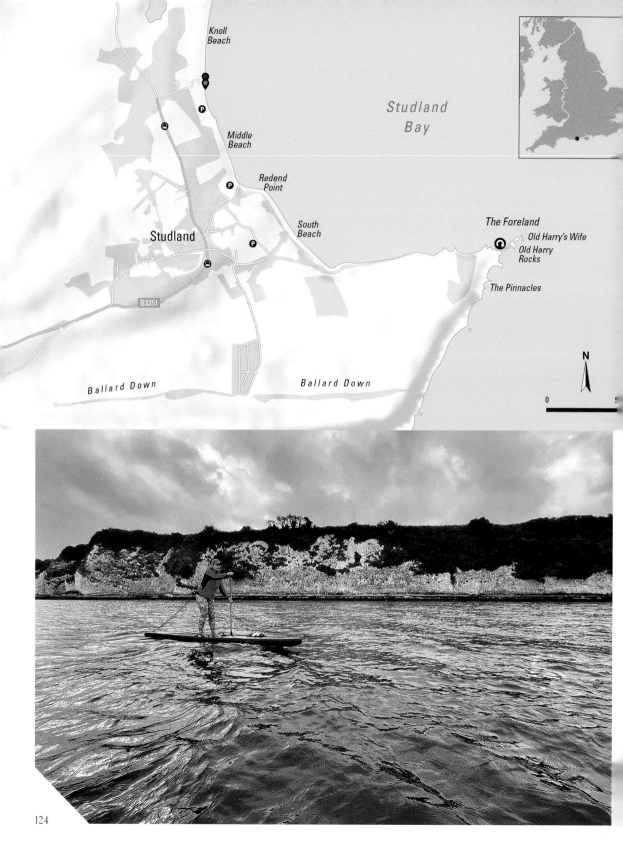

Knoll
Beach

Middle
Beach

Redend
Point

South
Beach

Studland

B3351

Studland
Bay

The Foreland
Old Harry's Wife
Old Harry
Rocks

The Pinnacles

N

0   5

Ballard Down   Ballard Down

Old Harry Rocks, Weymouth

EARLY STARTS, CHEERLEADING SUP FRIENDS, AWE-INSPIRING CLIFFS AND THE JOY OF SEAHORSES

'Lucy, Lucy, that's my swimsuit! I'd really like to wear it!'

It's 5.19 a.m. on a Monday morning and I am chasing a gorgeous chocolate springador around the bedroom. She's having such a lovely time playing with my costume that I can't help but laugh. That said, Lucy's owner Sarah Blues and I have a very special SUP adventure ahead and we really do need to be on the road before 6 a.m. Time, tide and winds wait for no paddleboarder.

Sarah has invited me to Weymouth to paddle to Old Harry Rocks, one of three chalk formations located at The Foreland or Handfast Point on the Isle of Purbeck in Dorset. The headland lies between the bays of Studland and Swanage, making it the most easterly point of the Jurassic Coast, a UNESCO World Heritage Site.

We had hoped to paddle here a few weeks beforehand but 60-kilometre-per-hour winds ruled it out. Sarah has been checking the forecast constantly and we have a plan: the winds are due to pick up around 10.30 a.m., so if we are on the water for 7.30 a.m. we can make it to Old Harry Rocks and be back safely on the beach in time. It's a five-kilometre-round trip from Middle Beach. We are both excited and have everything crossed that the forecast is right.

Sarah grew up respecting and learning about the sea. Her father was second coxswain for Weymouth RNLI and as a child she swam and pilot-gig rowed. By my bed she's kindly left *SUP Mag UK* and William Thomson's *The Book of Tides* to dip into. She only started paddleboarding a year ago, but her commitment to safety and sharing the benefits of the sea and SUP are already making a difference. Finding it difficult to buy well-fitting wetsuits and buoyancy aids, Sarah founded #PaddleKitHerWay, a campaign calling for companies to make paddleboarding kit more inclusive. With thorough research and great communication skills, she is already working with key brands and has encouraged many plus-size women to feel they belong on the water and to build their confidence and technical skills.

We will be paddling with Cherie, another powerhouse who recently discovered the joy of paddleboarding in Dorset. Having previously raced motorbikes, Cherie, who like me is in her late fifties, brings her competitive edge to the water and found herself on the podium at her first SUP race. They are each other's biggest cheerleaders and it feels such a privilege to launch from the beach in Studland Bay and head out to Old Harry Rocks together.

Studland Bay, which was designated a Marine Conservation Zone in 2019, is lined by six and a half kilometres of beaches. Knoll Beach is the largest and includes 900 metres designated as a naturist beach. There is also Shell Bay, Middle Beach and South Beach. With heathland, sand dune and wetland habitats, the area is home to the UK's six native reptiles. There is an ancient woodland and freshwater lake, known locally as Little Sea. In the National Trust shop I pick up a Sand Dune Safaris leaflet for visitors to record the birds, insects and plants they spot, and there is a lovely Nature Notes chalkboard for ideas of things to do and see.

We paddle into an inshore breeze, reminding each other that we will be flying back to the beach on our return, and cross

Opposite Cherie paddling near the limestone cliffs of Old Harry Rocks

the bay towards the bright orange buoys. My excitement rises as we get closer to Old Harry Rocks, and despite the slightly overcast day the limestone cliffs seem to glow. Old Harry and Old Harry's Wife were formed over thousands of years by coastal erosion of the cliff face, which initially created crevices, followed by caves and then arches. Ultimately, the arches collapsed, leaving chalk stacks. There is some debate about why they are called Old Harry: one story is that it is because the Devil once took a nap there, another that it's named after the fourteenth-century pirate Harry Paye from Poole, who used the rocks as cover before attacking passing merchant ships.

As we reach the headland, Sarah advises us to land on the beach so we can look at the water and decide if we want to paddle around. It is choppier at the point and on the Swanage side, so we choose to explore the beach instead. The light reflecting from the chalk is stunning. For a few minutes, I simply stand in awe at thousands of years of history before me, then turn to the sea anemones and limpets clinging to the rocks, grateful for the beauty we are fortunate to be witnessing.

Keenly aware of the time and forecast, we head back to our launch point, and with the wind behind our backs we do indeed zip along. Nearing the beach, Sarah tells me about the work of the Seahorse Trust to install environmentally friendly boat moorings

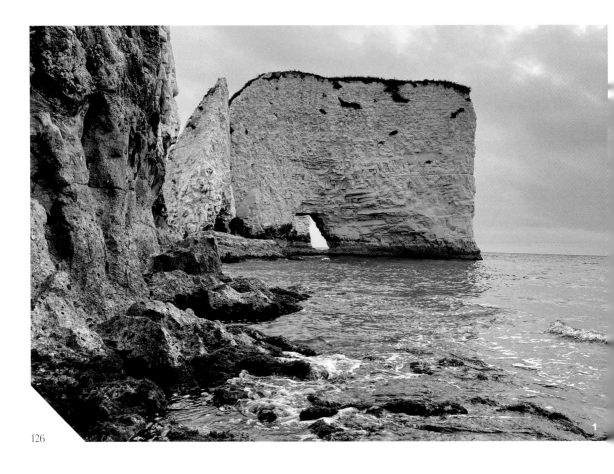

1

2 Sarah paddling at Studland Bay

to protect the seagrass and the increase in numbers of the protected spiny seahorses found in the bay. In summer 2020, during a single dive at Studland, 16 were recorded, including pregnant males and two babies.

A skein of geese fly overhead as we reach the shoreline and, once we have packed away our boards, we enjoy a delicious breakfast and hot chocolate at the National Trust cafe on Knoll Beach. The wind has begun to whip up as forecast and by the time we head home, presents from Dorset of course purchased, it would be too windy and choppy to paddle. Thanks to Sarah's meticulous planning, putting safety first and working as a team, we have enjoyed a gorgeous early morning on the water.

Old Harry Rocks and Studland Bay are stunning places to SUP and I am thrilled that we finally had chance to see them together.

As we leave I notice a sign that says the sand dunes are 'resting', asking visitors to use the footpaths. After a 5 a.m. start, a little rest sounds most appealing. Before that, however, Sarah and her partner Sid (and Lucy too of course) take me to the beautiful Isle of Portland to visit its red-and-white-striped lighthouse. They also point out the fast-moving Portland Race I've read about in *The Book of Tides*.

Sarah's SUP joy and SUP safety are always at the fore. Her family's RNLI heritage lives on, and for this I am truly grateful.

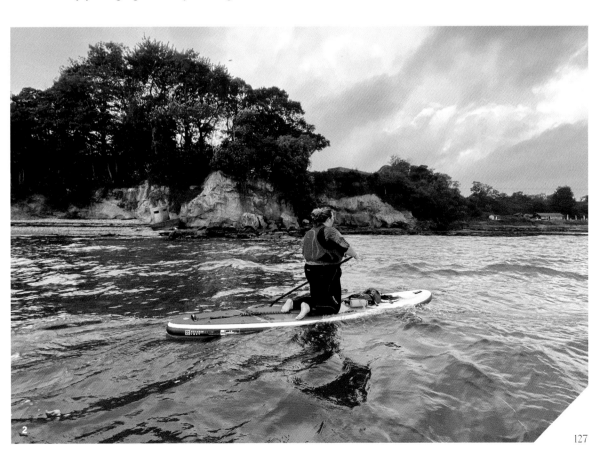

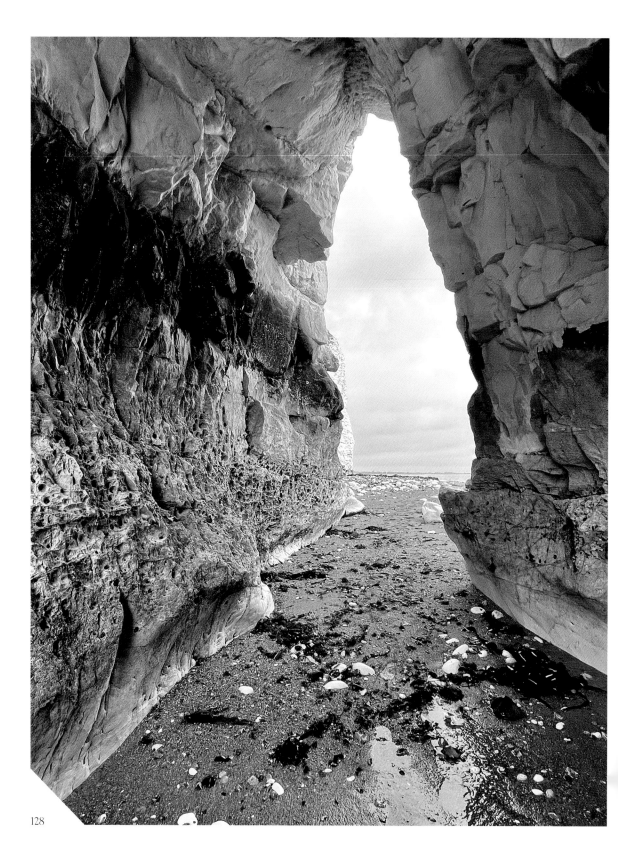

Technical information

DISTANCE **5km round trip.**

LAUNCH LOCATION
ENTRY AND EXIT POINT **SZ 034835/50.651, -1.953**
TURN AROUND POINT **SZ 054825/50.642, -1.924**

Difficulty

Paddleboarding experience is necessary for this trip and knowledge of wind and tides is important for Old Harry Rocks if you're going independently. The powerful forces which led to the formation of this landmark have also left traces below the surface of the water, which can combine with tides and conditions to make this a difficult place to paddle; expertise and knowledge are essential.

Paddleboarding close to the beaches would be a lovely alternative. Make sure you keep away from the safe swimming area that is cordoned off.

Getting there

Studland Bay is owned by the National Trust. The heritage Swanage railway has connections throughout Dorset on selected days, and from here frequent buses between Swanage and Bournemouth can take you to Studland Bay.

There is lots of pay-and-display car parking at Knoll Beach (SZ 034833/50.651, -1.953), Middle Beach (SZ 036829/50.645, -1.950), South Beach (SZ 038825/50.642, -1.948) and Shell Bay (SZ 035863/50.677, -1.951). Parking is free for National Trust members. The easiest car park to launch from is Knoll Beach. There is also a pay-and-display car park along Portland Beach Road (SY 669755/50.578, -2.469).

There are public toilets at South Beach and Middle Beach and an outdoor shower at Knoll Beach.

Route information

If you are visiting Weymouth, an alternative spot to launch is by Billy Winters Bar & Diner (a beach bar and diner on the beach), where you can paddle across the harbour to Sandsfoot Castle, a five-kilometre-round trip with small, hidden, sandy beaches along the route.

You will need to buy a permit to paddleboard here and you can buy one from Weymouth Watersports, which also offers instruction and tours, or 109 Watersports, which sells equipment.

Eating and drinking

» We had a delicious breakfast at the National Trust Cafe on Knoll Beach. There is also a gift shop and second-hand bookshop.

Instruction, guided tours and equipment hire

» Fore/Adventure offer paddleboarding lessons for beginners as well as guided tours to Old Harry Rocks for those with some experience. You can hire boards from them, but they can only be used if you stay less than 100m from the beach. You cannot take them to Old Harry Rocks. They also offer 'foraging and feasting' adventures and bushcraft skills as well as kayaking and coasteering.
» Josh the SUP Guide offers bespoke guided tours to nearby Lulworth Cove and Durdle Door and works with the team at Paddleboarding London.

Further information

» The Seahorse Trust:
  www.theseahorsetrust.org
» William Thomson, *The Book of Tides: A journey through the coastal waters of our island* (Quercus Publishing, 2016).

Opposite Peeking through a rock formation near Old Harry Rocks

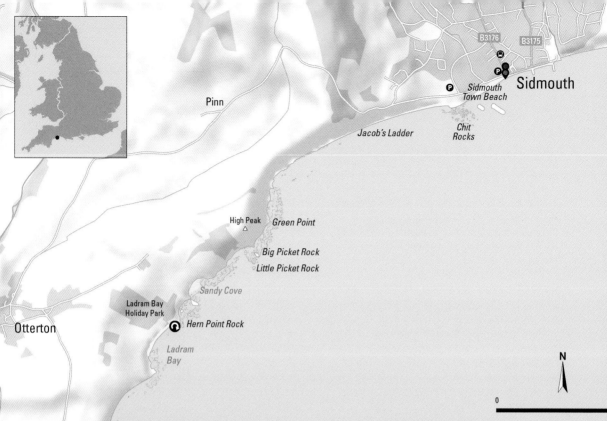

Pinn

B3176 B3175

Sidmouth
Town Beach

Sidmouth

Jacob's Ladder

Chit
Rocks

High Peak
△ Green Point

Big Picket Rock

Little Picket Rock

Sandy Cove

Ladram Bay
Holiday Park

Hern Point Rock

Otterton

Ladram
Bay

N

0

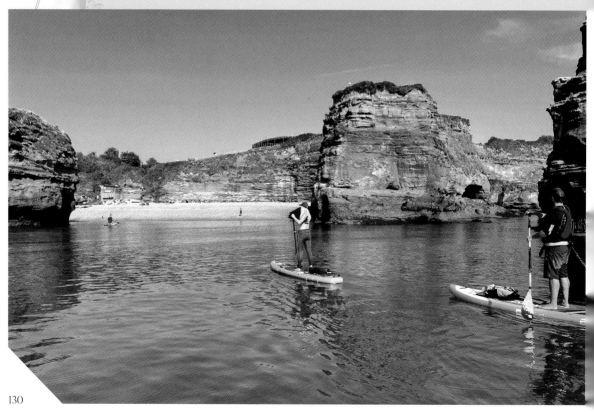

Sidmouth, East Devon

STRIPY DECKCHAIRS, RED CLIFFS, GLASSY WATERS AND LESSONS FROM THE WIND

'Proceed to the route. Proceed to the route.' It's the satnav on my phone reminding me that I have taken a wrong turn.

'I know, I know,' I reply, pulling over to check the map. I've arrived in Beer, a pretty village on the East Devon coast, after a long journey from Yorkshire, accompanied by inspiring paddleboarding podcasts from *SUP Hub NI* and *SUPfm*.

Struggling to find somewhere to stay, with my romantic dream of 'van life, travelling and writing' cut short by financial reality, I turned to my friends at Beer Women's Institute for help, asking the president if perhaps someone in their WI runs a B & B.

'I'm not a B & B but you'd be very welcome to stay with me,' came a lovely reply from one of their members, Penny. And so a few minutes later I finally arrive at her doorstep, and in true WI style am welcomed in and offered a nice cup of tea. Penny's gorgeous home will be my base for the next two days as I explore some of Devon's paddleboarding spots, including a coastal journey from Sidmouth, a sunset SUP on the River Exe (p137), a windy paddle along the Exeter Ship Canal (p137) and on to Salcombe (p143).

I'm keen to see Beer's beautiful shingle beach, sheltered by white, chalk cliffs and home to a working fishing fleet. There are pink and blue beach huts and stripy deckchairs to rent, dippers in the sea and friends enjoying picnics in the evening sun. I wander through the village to Jimmy Green Marine, my dad's favourite chandlery, and pass pubs, galleries and allotments perched on the clifftop. Tomorrow it's an early start for Sidmouth,

a town just over 12 kilometres west.

Like Beer, Sidmouth lies along the UNESCO-World-Heritage Jurassic Coast and is part of East Devon's Area of Outstanding Natural Beauty. It's nestled within the lush, green hills and woods of the Sid Valley at the mouth of the River Sid. Originally a fishing village, it became a popular holiday destination in the eighteenth and nineteenth centuries, with the elegant Regency buildings, now hotels and restaurants, lining the promenade along the town front.

It has two beaches: Sidmouth Town Beach, where we launch, and to the west Jacob's Ladder, so called because of the set of white steps that lead from the beach to Connaught Gardens, opened in 1934. You can also reach the South West Coast Path, which at 986 kilometres is one of the UK's longest national trails. It starts in Minehead in Somerset, follows the coastline of Cornwall, Devon and Dorset and finishes at Poole Harbour.

Sidmouth is also known for the deep-red cliffs that flank the town. Dating back over 235 million years to the Triassic period, they provide the stunning backdrop to our paddle today. You can see some of the reptile fossils found in the cliffs' Otter Sandstone as well as learn more about the town's history at the lovely Sidmouth Museum on Church Street, which I later visit.

The tide is in and there's a slight morning mist as I arrive. Dog walkers and runners are enjoying the kilometre-and-a-half-long esplanade along the main beach. The sea is calm and the sun's glittery paths surround the swimmers in the sea as the waves gently lap on the shingle beach. I am here to meet Becky Dickinson, surfer, rambler and paddleboarder

Opposite Mike and Becky arriving at Ladram Bay

131

who writes about her Devon and Cornwall adventures. We will be joined by Mike Smith, freelance SUP instructor, river guide and father to Lilly, who also offers free paddleboarding sessions to teenagers to support their mental health in his SUP-Planet Earth role. Becky has been carefully watching the weather and with high winds forecast for tomorrow, today is the day for the coast.

We park in the private car park opposite Sidmouth Town Beach and launch. Our destination is Ladram Bay, about four kilometres south-west towards Budleigh Salterton. The sun is burning the sea mist and the skies are a bright blue as we paddle along, passing Jacob's Ladder. The magnificent red cliffs and trees along the South West Coast Path are reflected in the glassy sea. Suddenly there is a loud crash

and looking back we spot dust rising where rocks have tumbled down from the cliff face. It's a timely reminder why this part of the beach is closed to walkers and how fortunate we are as paddleboarders to have such a stunning view of the Jurassic Coast. Shoals of small fish swim under and in front of our boards and cormorants are drying their wings on the rocks as we make our way to the towering stacks ahead, some of the most magnificent and well known along the East Devon coastline. They are the remains of caves and arches that have been eroded over time, collapsing into the sea and leaving these stumps.

We have now reached Ladram Bay, a privately owned beach, part of the Ladram Bay Holiday Park. Carrying our boards safely on to the pebbles, we take a moment for a drink and

1

1 Arriving back at Sidmouth **2** Soaking up the view

ice cream, soaking up the sun. It's time to return to Sidmouth and cherish what must be one of the calmest paddle trips I've ever experienced. These are the moments when you feel you are walking on water, and what a privilege they are.

As we reach Sidmouth the tide is now on its way out and, sitting on our boards with our legs dangling in the warm sea, we paddle around the breakwaters that protect the shore from the waves. There are paddleboarders enjoying the sunshine and children splashing in the shallow waters close to the beach. With everything packed away, Becky gives us a tour of the town before a delicious lunch from The Bagel Shop, where we arrange our next paddle.

Her planning has been spot on, as we have enjoyed glassy, calm waters. The next day on my way back from the Exeter Ship Canal (p137)

I pop to Branscombe, which lies between Sidmouth and Beer. Despite blue skies and sunshine, the wind is up and the waves are rolling noisily on to the beach. I meet a couple of local chaps with their boards.

'How was it?' I ask. 'A bit like paddling hard and getting nowhere?'

'That's about right!' they laughed.

They had been safe and within their limits, but it was a very different paddle to the day before. It reminds me of two important SUP lessons: one is that watching the wind and tides is hugely important for coastal paddling, and the second is that if the sea and forecast are calm and glassy and you have the opportunity, seize it, because you never quite know what tomorrow will bring. Stay glassy, friends!

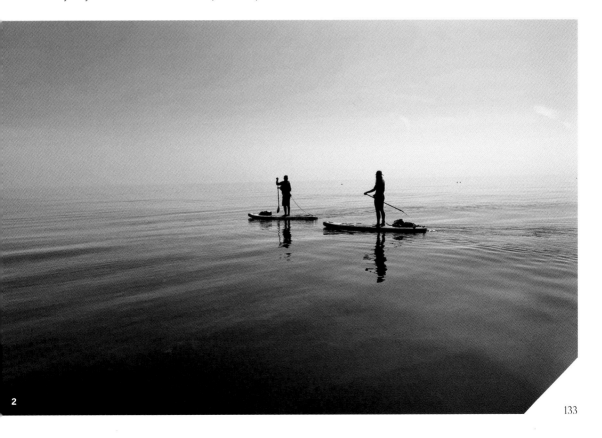

Technical information

DISTANCE **10km round trip.**

LAUNCH LOCATION
ENTRY AND EXIT POINT **SY 125871/50.677, -3.240**
TURN AROUND POINT **SY 097851/50.659, -3.278**

Difficulty

Paddleboarding along the coast requires an understanding of tides and wind if going independently. Paddleboarding close to the beach would be lovely.

Getting there

The nearest railway station is Honiton, which has direct connections to Exeter and London, and from here you can catch a bus to Sidmouth. Buses to Exeter also stop a few hundred metres from Sidmouth Town Beach.

Bedford Lawn car park is across the road from the beach (SY 124872/50.678, -3.240). This is a private car park where you pay at the gate, and if you stay longer than expected you simply pay extra.

Route information

Sidmouth's independent lifeboat has lifeguards on the beach in the summer.

Sidmouth Town Council has a webcam on the Esplanade.

Route information

Ladram Bay Holiday Park is happy for you to land on the beach and enjoy something to eat and drink at its cafes/shop. However, parking and launching at the site is only available to guests who stay there. You could take your own picnic and enjoy it on your board on the trip.

Eating and drinking

- » There are lots of places to eat in Sidmouth and many ice cream parlours.
- » The Bagel Shop serves delicious bagels and drinks.
- » I bought picnic things for the journey at the refill shop Fillfull.

Instruction, guided tours and equipment

- » Mike Smith offers SUP instruction and paddleboarding sessions for teenagers for their mental health at SUP-Planet Earth.
- » Jurassic Paddle Sports is based on Sidmouth Town Beach and offers paddleboard hire, one-on-one coaching and water safety sessions.

Further information

- » Becky Dickinson's SUP Becks blog: *www.supbecks.com*
- » OneWave Sidmouth is a non-profit surfing and paddleboarding community offering SUP meetings for mental health on Sidmouth Town Beach: *www.facebook. com/OneWaveSidmouth*

Opposite Admiring Sidmouth's red cliffs © Becky Dickinson, @beachy_becks

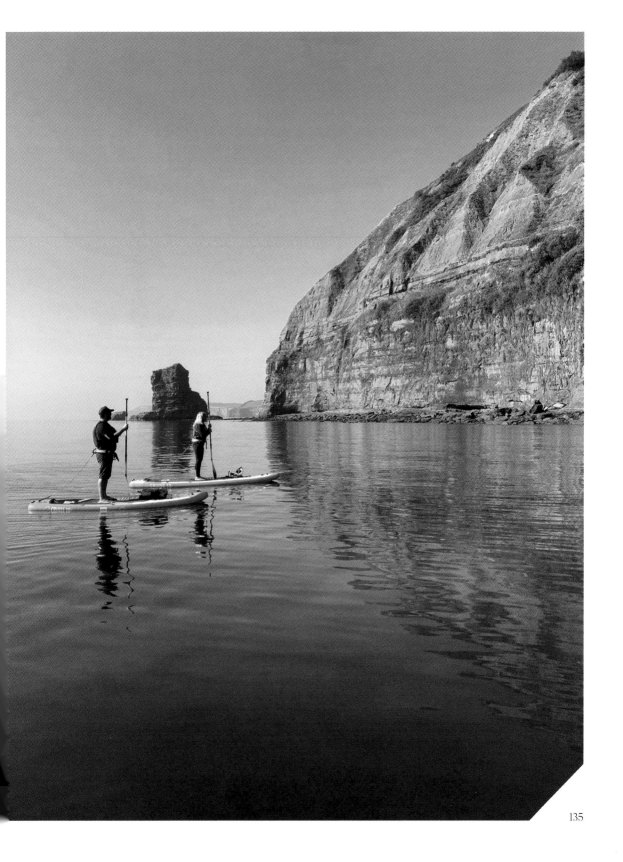

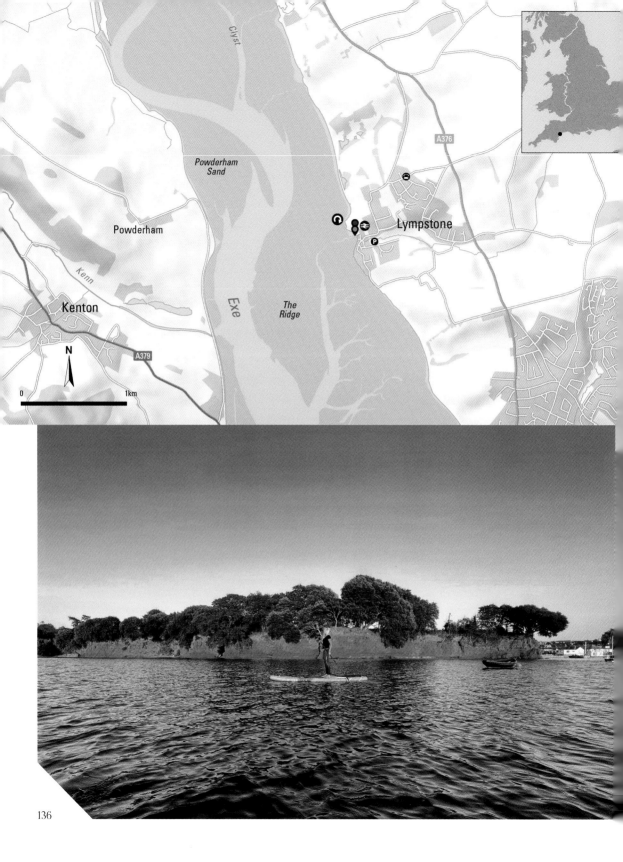

River Exe and Exeter Ship Canal

WASHING LINES ON THE FORESHORE, SUNSET AT LYMPSTONE, A PADDLE TO THE PUB AND WHOOSHING TO THE QUAYSIDE

Pink and yellow tops hang neatly on the washing lines between poles along the foreshore as the evening sun sparkles on the estuary behind them. Three swans glide serenely across the gentle waves and a skein of geese fly above. There's a dog swimming enthusiastically in the warm waters, closely followed by his owner, who is smiling broadly. Sailing boats sway gently on their moorings. The roar of a Great Western Railway train hurtling past on the opposite bank momentarily drowns out the laughter of a group of paddleboarders. Kayakers launch from the slip. On the bench beneath Peter's Tower, built by William Peters in 1885 in memory of his wife, friends are chatting with a glass in their hand and a picnic by their side, their faces bathed in the sunshine as they sit watching the horizon, as if waiting for a show to begin.

Becky Dickinson and I are in Lympstone, a village on the east side of Devon's River Exe, just after high tide, and the show we have come to see is the sun setting behind the hills in the distance. After our glassy paddle from Sidmouth to Ladram Bay (p131), we arranged an evening SUP on the estuary. I explore Budleigh Salterton Beach and then meet Becky at The Swan Inn for tea. We make our way through the narrow, cobbled alleyways, under the washing line and on to the water, heading northwards towards Topsham. The stunning red sandstone of the cliffs and the trees above glow. Round the corner a couple with a Thermos flask and mugs squeeze on to a tiny bit of beach that

will grow bigger as the tide recedes from the estuary. Mike Smith, with whom we spent the morning in Sidmouth, has joined us from Exmouth with friends and will return on the outgoing tide.

The River Exe rises on Exmoor National Park in Somerset and flows around 80 kilometres across moorland and through Exeter, reaching the English Channel at Exmouth. The section of the Exe Estuary where the sea meets the freshwater river starts south of Exeter, and Topsham, Exton, Lympstone, Dawlish Warren, Starcross and Cockwood lie along its banks. The estuary is an important site for birds and wildlife, and is made up of five different types of habitat: mudflats, eel grass, mussel beds, saltmarsh and reed beds. It is home to many species of snails, worms and clams that attract the wading birds that feed on them, such as avocets, oystercatchers, grey plover and black-tailed godwits.

We stand quietly on our boards watching the sun as it finally disappears behind the horizon, then return to the village, glancing back momentarily for one last look as the joyful sound of band practice fills the air on Chapel Road. We have been on the estuary for just under an hour and paddled just over a kilometre and a half, and yet it has been quite magical. For me this is one of the beauties of paddleboarding: there is no narrative that says we *have* to achieve a certain distance, time or speed. If we wish to, of course we can. We can also simply *be* on the water, treasuring the moment, belonging, if only for an evening, to a community and experiencing somewhere new. We can choose to paddle hard one day and

Opposite Stunning red sandstone cliffs near Lympstone

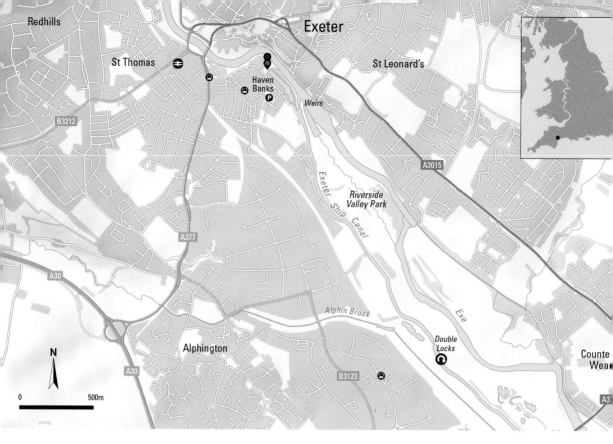

pause to watch the sunset another. It's all SUP. It's the happiness it brings and what it means to you that matters.

The next morning I meet Becky at Exeter Quayside to paddle along the Exeter Ship Canal. The wind has picked up as forecast and the canal will offer some shelter that we would not have on the sea. Old warehouses and cellars converted into shops and cafes are already buzzing as friends and families enjoy the sunshine. Both the River Exe and the Exeter Ship Canal pass through the quayside and run parallel to each other heading south.

We launch at the pontoon next to AS Watersports and set off into the breeze, passing a few sailing boats and further along two interesting, larger, rusty boats that appear to have been abandoned for some time. Within minutes we are into lush countryside, with trees and reeds lining the towpath. It feels and looks different to other canals I've paddled along and a little research explains why: the canal is in fact one of the oldest artificial waterways in the UK,

built in the 1560s to bypass two weirs along the River Exe that had blocked trading ships from easily reaching the port in Exeter. The Countess Wear area of Exeter was named after the Countess of Devon, Isabella de Fortibus, who built the canal around the 1270s in order to divert the river to power her mills. Construction from 1566 meant it was a long time before the canals were expanded during the Industrial Revolution, such as the Leeds and Liverpool in the north. Like others around the country, the introduction of the railways heralded the decline of the canals as a means of transport and trade. Today it is mainly used by canoeists, kayakers and paddleboarders and enjoyed by cyclists and walkers along the towpath.

The canal is just over eight kilometres long and has two locks: the Double Locks and, further along, the tidal Turf Lock at the end of the canal, linking it to the River Exe. The pub here, The Turf, has no car parking and can only be reached by bike or on foot, or alternatively by water, which is an idea for another day.

Our destination today is the Double Locks pub, two and a half kilometres from the quayside. We paddle along in the warmth of the sun, ducking under the swing bridges and navigating around groups of teenagers laughing in canoes and kayaks. There are children cooling off with a dip in the water and swans gliding past nonchalantly. The pub is quiet today and has plenty of room on the decking by the canal, so we exit just before the lock and carry our boards to the table, passing an upcycled red telephone box.

After a lovely lunch we return to Exeter, this time with the wind behind our backs which makes it a much faster journey. Coming into the quayside, Becky and I put our paddles out to the side, creating a sail, and whoosh along with the wind, passing the boats on the water and on the dock. It's a joy to see other paddleboarders sailing along, smiling together as we experience the same sense of freedom.

I later realise this has been another first for me: paddleboarding to a pub for lunch and back. This is something I know many SUP social groups and my friends at the Paddle Cabin on the River Medway in Kent enjoy together. I imagine this trip would be beautiful on a crisp autumn or winter's day if you wrap up warm. Maybe take a flask and enjoy a hot chocolate or breakfast from the Boatyard Bakery on your board. For a longer adventure, you could paddle to the end of the canal at Turf Lock and return or go down the River Exe (check the tides and watch out for your fin) and return on the canal.

There are so many possibilities for happy paddleboarding on the River Exe and Exeter Ship Canal, from a magical sunset SUP to a relaxed lunch on the canal, or setting yourself a longer adventure to explore the estuary from River Exe. From Exeter Quayside you are in the city one minute and the country the next. Whatever you choose, however quickly or far you go, I hope you'll return richer for the experiences, as I did.

Technical information

DISTANCE
LYMPSTONE **1.6km round trip.**
EXETER SHIP CANAL **5km round trip.**

....

LAUNCH LOCATION
LYMPSTONE
ENTRY AND EXIT POINT **SX 988841/50.648, -3.432**
TURN AROUND POINT **SX 987842/50.649, -3.435**
EXETER SHIP CANAL
ENTRY AND EXIT POINT **SX 921920/50.717, -3.530**
TURN AROUND POINT **SX 932900/50.700, -3.513**

Difficulty

Paddleboarding at Lympstone requires an understanding of tides and wind if you're going independently. The best time to go would be one to two hours before high tide.

Paddleboarding on the Exeter Ship Canal is sheltered and a good spot for beginners. Watch out for moorings and other boats using the canal.

Getting there

Lympstone

There is a railway station at Lympstone with connections to Exmouth, less than 200m from the shoreline.

Buses between Exeter St Davids station and Exmouth stop in Lympstone, just under a kilometre from the launch point.

There is a pay-and-display car park in the village at Underhill car park (SX 990840/50.647, -3.430). There are public toilets in the car park.

Exeter Ship Canal

Exeter Central railway station, with connections to Exmouth and London, is just over a kilometre from the quayside. Buses throughout Exeter stop a few hundred metres from the launch point. National Express travels to Exeter from major cities across Britain, including London.

There is a pay-and-display car park near the Haven Banks car park (SX 921917/50.715, -3.530). There are public toilets on the quayside.

Route information

Lympstone
Launch from the slipway by Peter's Tower. To launch from the harbour slipway you need to be a member.

Exeter Ship Canal
Launch from the pontoon at the start of the canal. This is owned by AS Watersports. However, they are happy for you to use it if you ensure you respect other users and do not leave anything on the pontoon.

Eating and drinking
» We had a lovely meal at The Swan Inn in Lympstone.
» Boatyard Bakery sells hot drinks, bread and baked goods.
» Veg Box Cafe serves plant-based breakfasts and lunch, American pancakes and smoothies.
» We had a lovely lunch at the Double Locks pub in Exeter.

Instruction, guided tours and equipment
» Exmouth Watersports in Exmouth offers paddleboard tuition and hire.
» Edge Watersports offers paddleboard hire, tuition and guided tours from Exmouth.
» AS Watersports on Exeter Quayside offers tuition, SUP socials and paddleboard hire. It also has a retail shop with an extensive range of paddleboards and kit to buy. Its website has a link to different routes to take on the Exeter Ship Canal and River Exe. Remember to check the tides so there is enough water for the journey and your fin. Go down on the river and return on the canal.
» Saddles and Paddles offers paddleboard hire.

Further information
» AS Watersports has a helpful map on where to paddle in the area: *www.aswatersports.co.uk*

1 Exeter Ship Canal 2 Exeter Quayside 3 Glimpsing Lympstone from the water
4 Red sandstone cliffs by Lympstone 5 A shared paddleboard at sunset in Lympstone

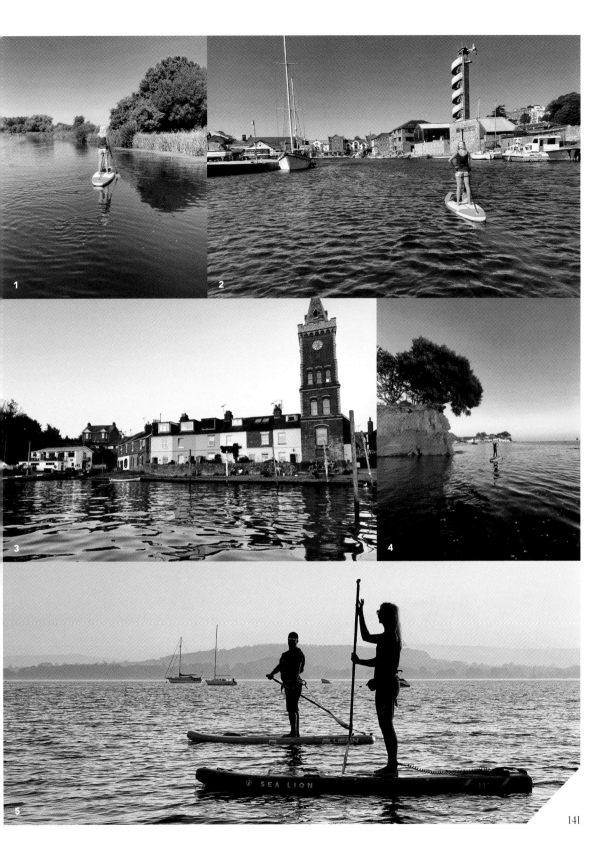

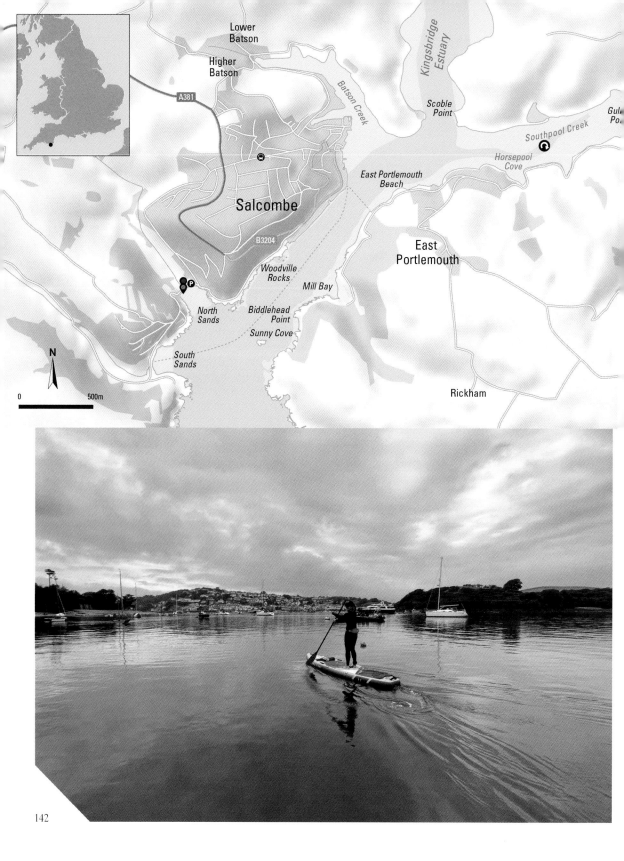

Salcombe

BEING YOUR OWN SUNSHINE ON A RAINY DAY, EXPLORING CREEKS, HARBOUR LIFE AND PICNICS ON THE BEACH

'Hmm, the weather isn't looking great,' says Penny, my lovely WI friend, as we're having breakfast in Beer, 'I hope it's OK for you in Salcombe today.'

'I know, it really isn't,' I agree, trying to remain optimistic despite the forecast of heavy rain. Grateful for the sunshine I've enjoyed in East Devon over the last couple of days, the outlook is decidedly greyer and wetter for the rest of the week as I move on to South Devon and Cornwall.

A couple of hours later and the heavens open as I make my way down a very narrow lane to North Sands, at the mouth of the Salcombe-Kingsbridge Estuary. Living on the edge of the Yorkshire Dales, I'm used to squeezing into passing spaces and hedges to let cars go by and I'm *definitely* used to the rain. Today, however, on unfamiliar roads, with potholes and construction traffic at every turn, it all feels overwhelming.

I've come to spend the day with Jojo O'Brien, founder of Wildbeings, who offers outdoor fitness retreats to nourish her clients' physical, emotional and mental well-being. A ski instructor for over 20 years who is also qualified in paddleboarding, open-water swimming and water rescue, Jojo has an irrepressible enthusiasm for life. She is perhaps the only person I know who, on our first meeting, asks if I'd like to go for a walk in the pouring rain. I later learn this is something she regularly offers her retreat clients, and they love it! Her cheery disposition is infectious and I suggest she jumps in the car and tells me more about Salcombe and her work.

Salcombe is a popular seaside town and harbour which sits at the most southerly tip of Devon, within the South Devon Area of Outstanding Natural Beauty. The Salcombe-Kingsbridge Estuary, where the freshwater meets the sea, is a Site of Special Scientific Interest, a Local Nature Reserve and part of the South Devon Heritage Coast. The estuary is unusual as it is not fed by one large river but by a number of smaller streams, including Frogmore, Bowcombe, Batson, East Allington and Sherford. There are reed beds, mudflats and eelgrass beds, and the worms and snails found in the mudflats make it an important feeding area for wading birds and fish populations. According to the Seahorse Trust, it is also a safe haven for both the spiny and short-snouted seahorse.

As we peer out of the car a little while later the rain has stopped, and while it is by no means the turquoise waters and blue skies I had hoped to share with you, the sea is calm and there's no wind.

'Let's go for it!' we say in unison, and within a few minutes we are launching from the flat, sandy North Sands. To our right is South Sands, another pretty, sheltered cove with a cafe, two hotels and paddleboard hire. The cove is overlooked by the nearby National Trust's beautiful Overbeck's Gardens. Described by the trust as a 'sub-tropical garden paradise' with 'unusual plants from all around the globe', the garden is possible because of Salcombe's mild microclimate; it includes a date palm, orange and lemon trees and a magnolia collection from the Himalaya planted in 1901.

We paddle out to Sunny Cove on the opposite East Portlemouth side of the estuary and through the rocks exposed by the outgoing tide,

Opposite Jojo facing Salcombe

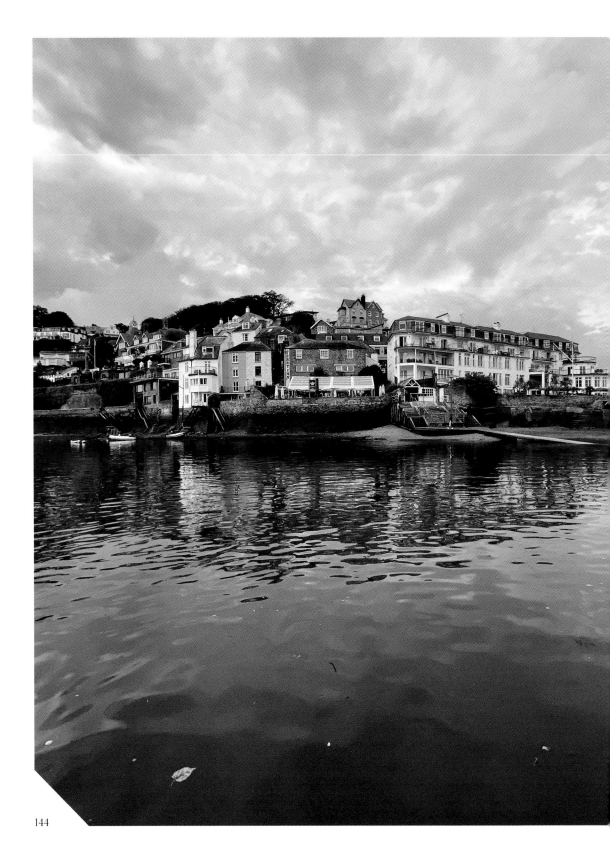

looking down at the seaweed and pools beneath. The South West Coast Path, from Minehead in Somerset through Devon and Cornwall to Poole in Dorset, runs through the trees above. I breathe in deeply, exhaling the stresses of the journey, realising how much calmer I am now we are on the water and the earlier dramas float away into the sea. I also remind myself to 'paddle the paddle I'm paddling', no comparison to photos, hopes or expectations of what it should be like. I take a moment to reflect how fortunate I am to be here; it's time to bring some sunshine of my own to the day as we make our way past beautiful Mill Bay and Small's Cove beaches.

Salcombe Harbour, especially during the height of the summer season, is a very busy place for boats. While today it is quieter, we paddle cautiously, keeping a good distance from the moorings and looking out for the South Sands Ferry and other crafts moving through the water. Jojo's advice is to paddle on either side of the estuary rather than down the middle of the channel: 'this is for safety and there's always something new to see, it's really magical,' she says. Her favourite times are between 7 a.m. and 11 a.m. before there's too much activity on the water. The sea breeze can pick up during the day in the summer, but often calms down after 6 p.m., offering glassy, flat conditions.

As we paddle along, we can hear the tinkling of bells and see bunting and flags fluttering in the wind. We look up at the white, blue and pink buildings that are hotels and homes in the town, wave to people sitting outside the restaurants and find a spot to pull up by the slipway to go ashore. It's time to treat ourselves to lunch from The Salcombe Yawl, and I go for a wander through the bustling town. Then we are back on our boards, quietly watching a heron nearby, for a paddle past

The Baltic Exchange III, the RNLI's Tamar-class, all-weather lifeboat, and back over to East Portlemouth Beach. We find a comfy spot on the sand with the most beautiful views across the harbour and to Snapes Point, enjoy our sandwiches and chat.

From here Jojo points out the different creeks leading north that she has enjoyed exploring, including Batson ('very *Swallows and Amazons*,' she says), Kingsbridge, Southpool and Waterhead creeks. On sunny days, or cold winter days with a picnic, she enjoys running, hiking, paddleboarding and swimming with friends, family and her clients. Wildbeings isn't just her work, it's how she lives her life, and I feel inspired listening to her.

We paddle along Southpool Creek, admiring the boats and their reflection in the calm, glassy water and then return through the harbour and head to North Sands. The wind begins to pick up so we need to dig a little deeper and paddle a little harder, saying hello to a friend of Jojo's sailing nearby.

After 12 kilometres on the estuary, we arrive back at Fort Charles and float past the spaghetti-like seaweed. Salcombe has been a joy, and with an understanding of the tides and wind in the estuary it offers so many different beaches and creeks to explore on your paddleboard. Leaving North Sands, I reflect upon what Nikki Peterson, coach at *Psychologies* magazine, charity CEO and paddleboarder once wrote to me about SUP: '[it] offers peace, quiet, tranquility and time to think. When I paddle, the usual noise and clutter that occupies my headspace disappears. I always come off the water feeling like my body and soul have had a full cup of nourishment.'

A day in South Devon with Jojo O'Brien has definitely been a cup of nourishment. As I head to Plymouth en route to my next SUP trip, I am deeply grateful that my cup is so full.

Opposite Salcombe Harbour

1 Exposed rocks at Sunny Cove

Technical information

DISTANCE **12km round trip.**

LAUNCH LOCATION
ENTRY POINT **SX 731382/50.230, -3.781**
TURN AROUND POINT **SX 755391/50.239, -3.747**

ALTERNATIVE ROUTE **You could have a lovely time paddleboarding close to the shore in North Sands Bay and South Sands Bay.**

Difficulty

Paddleboarding through the estuary, harbour and creeks requires an understanding of the tides and wind if you're going independently. To explore the creeks, Jojo recommends going up an hour before high tide and then returning on the outgoing tide, otherwise you may find yourself on the mudflats, which is not good for you or the birds that feed there. Returning to North Sands on an outgoing tide, cross to the Fort Charles side of the estuary after the harbour.

Getting there

The nearest railway station is Totnes, with connections to Plymouth, London, Cardiff and Aberdeen. Buses from Totnes to Salcombe stop a kilometre and a half away from the launch point in Salcombe.

Be aware that a satnav may take you down the narrowest of lanes. Use the route that takes you via Sandhills Road. There is a pay-and-display at North Sands (SX 730382/50.230, -3.782). There are public toilets a few hundred metres from the car park, up the hill to the east of the beach.

Route information

Salcombe Harbour Authority charges an annual fee of £6 to paddle in the harbour and Salcombe-Kingsbridge Estuary. You can visit

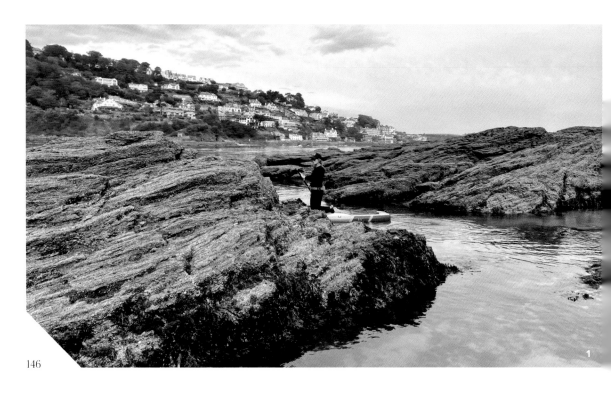

1

2 Passing Mill Bay

the harbour office on the day or complete the registration form on its website in advance and the licence will be posted to you. There is no daily/weekly rate, it is a £6 flat fee.

Eating and drinking

» There are lots of places to eat in Salcombe. The Salcombe Yawl is just by the slip on Batson Creek, selling sandwiches, drinks and cakes.
» The Winking Prawn at North Sands serves salads and sandwiches and is also a beach shop.

Instruction, guided tours and equipment

» Jojo O'Brien's Wildbeings offers paddleboarding morning and evening sessions from North Sands, as well as wellness days and retreats and outdoor fitness classes.

» North Sands Water Sports offers mobile paddleboard hire and sales. They will drop the boards at your accommodation or meet you at North Sands.
» Sea Kayak Salcombe offers paddleboard hire from South Sands.
» Salcombe Paddleboarding offers tuition, guided tours and paddleboard hire from Port Waterhouse in East Portlemouth, which is along the estuary and opposite Salcombe town centre.
» Salcombe Boats & Boards offers paddleboard hire from Salcombe town centre.

Further information

» The Seahorse Trust: *www.theseahorsetrust.org*

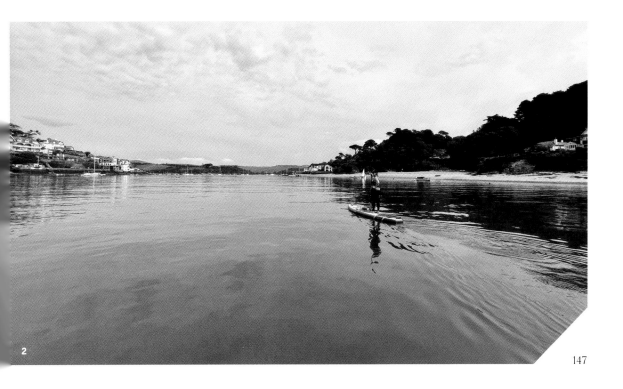

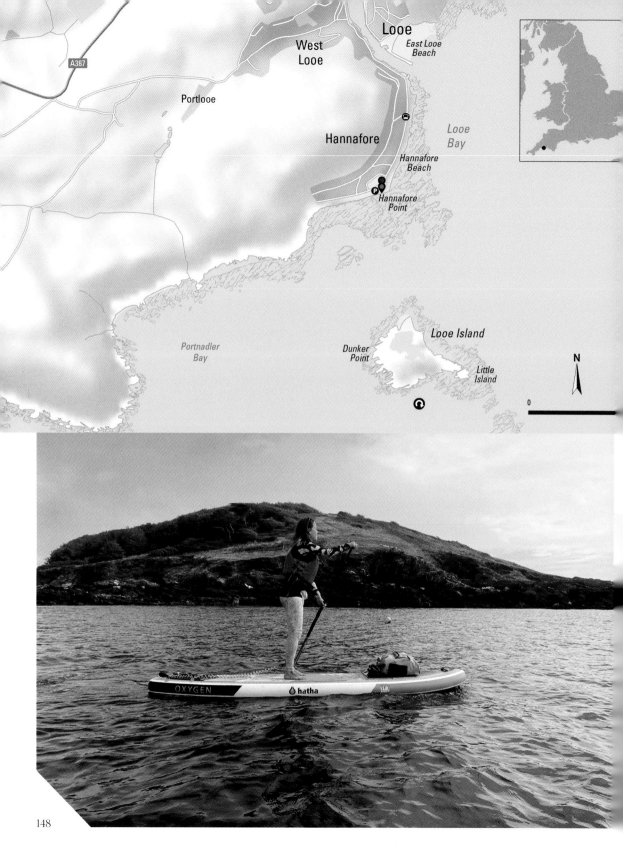

West
Looe

East Looe
Beach

Portlooe

Hannafore

Looe
Bay

Hannafore
Beach

Hannafore
Point

Portnadler
Bay

Dunker
Point

Looe Island

Little
Island

N

0

OXYGEN   🜁 hatha

Looe Island and Mullion Cove

TWO SISTERS BUY AN ISLAND, A #2MINUTEBEACHCLEAN BOARD, DRAMATIC CLIFFS ON THE LIZARD PENINSULA AND BEING GUESTS ON THE OCEAN

I turn for one final look at the sea in the distance. The late summer light is fading and I really must hurry to the car or I'll be changing and deflating my board in the dark. This has been such an extraordinary paddle at Cornwall's Mullion Cove; I want to savour the moment for as long as I can. The excited cries of children jumping into the sea from the harbour wall carry across the houses as the sun sets on the horizon. I close my eyes and breathe in the sea air. 'What an adventure we've had, Grace'. I whisper to my board.

My time with Steph Barnicoat, founder of SUP with Steph, marine biologist and author, has been bookended by the magic of Cornish islands. We began at Looe Island, a marine nature reserve in the English Channel, about a kilometre and a half from the harbour town of Looe. We finished here at Mullion Cove, 85 kilometres away from Looe, on the Lizard peninsula, around 11 kilometres from Lizard Point, the most southerly point on mainland Britain. Beautiful, wild and precious, they have taught me once again what a privilege it is to be a paddleboarder and the responsibility we have to look after the oceans, marine mammals and birdlife we are fortunate enough to see.

'Just watch your step on the seaweed,' cautions Steph a couple of days before, as we make our way across the rock pools and launch from Hannafore Beach, a long stretch of shingly coastline. The sky is blue, although clouds are gathering as we paddle towards Looe Island's west shore.

Steph has been fascinated by the ocean since childhood. She went on to study marine biology and now specialises in marine mammal bioacoustics. She volunteers with a local 'Your Shore' group affiliated to the Cornwall Wildlife Trust and is a marine mammal medic for British Diver Marine Life Rescue.

Looe Island is a 22.5-acre nature reserve; it is part of the Whitsand and Looe Bay Marine Conservation Zone and is owned and managed by the Cornwall Wildlife Trust. It is home to many nesting birds such as cormorants, shags and oystercatchers and hosts one of Cornwall's most significant breeding colonies of the great black-backed gull. The island has a sycamore woodland, a flock of Hebridean sheep, many species of butterflies and grey seal visitors that the wardens and volunteers from the Cornwall Seal Group Research Trust are surveying and identifying.

The island was bequeathed to the Cornwall Wildlife Trust by Roselyn 'Babs' Atkins upon her death, aged 86, in 2004. Babs and her sister Evelyn 'Attie' Atkins, originally from Epsom in Surrey, had fulfilled their lifelong dream to live on an island together when they purchased it in 1965. Evelyn wrote two charming books about their life, which I have read, called *We Bought an Island* and *Tales From Our Cornish Island*.

The trust hosts special visits to the reserve and the home where Babs and Attie lived, but otherwise no one is permitted to land, by foot, boat or SUP, as they want to preserve its habitat and tranquility. If you can't visit for an organised tour, you can read the fascinating blog the warden shares about her work, including details on 'the teeny weeny stuff', 'the greeny stuff', 'the feathery stuff' and 'the salty stuff'.

I feel deeply grateful to paddle along, spotting the sheep grazing above and the

Opposite Passing Looe Island

149

gulls perched on the jagged reefs, keeping far enough away that we don't disturb them. In the distance we notice a seal raise its head as it rests on an outcrop near the island. We aren't sure if it has seen us, the kayakers that are paddling a little further out or the orange rigid inflatable boat (RIB) that just sped past. All we know is that it is now alert.

'Do you mind if we go back the way we've come rather than go round the island as planned?' asks Steph. 'Time hauled out for seals is so important and I don't want to add any stress to the seal.'

'Of course,' I reply. We paddle away quietly and slowly, turning to check on the seal, which is once again back to resting on the rock in peace.

The wind picks up and for a few moments we whoosh along, holding our paddles to the side so they become sails. We pass along the eastern shore of the island, where the Island House and Smuggler's Cottage sit, then return to the beach past the spaghetti-like seaweed and mast of an old boat lodged within the rock pools. I take a moment for a litter pick then pop to the Island View Cafe for some chocolate flapjack and chat about the #2MinuteBeachClean station they look after. Today has been a magical start to my time in Cornwall.

'Wow, just wow,' I gasp, looking up at the huge rock stacks above as we leave the protection of the harbour walls and paddle out. It's a late summer evening a couple of days later and the sun is setting on the horizon. Ahead lies Mullion Island, also known as Toldhu, and to our left and right are the cliffs and caves of Mullion Cove, nestled on the west coast of the Lizard peninsula, an Area of Outstanding Natural Beauty. My research had shown photos of the nature reserve as turquoise seas and a small pebbly beach. Now, from the water the dark, volcanic rocks tower above and lumpy waves hit the cliff face. What stories these caves could tell about smugglers of the past, I wonder?

Mullion Island, which lies just under a kilometre ahead of us, is owned by the National Trust and is part of a local Site of Specific Scientific Interest. Like Looe Island, it is an important breeding colony for great black-backed gulls, guillemots, shags and cormorants, and public access is prohibited.

In 2019, wardens who monitor the site noticed thousands of elastic bands on the island and were initially confused as to how they could have reached such a remote spot. The conclusion was that, over many years, the gulls had fed on the bands in the commercial flower fields on the mainland, mistaking them for worms, and then regurgitated them. It is sobering to read that herring gull populations, vocal as they are individually, are actually on the decline.

'Do you want to paddle closer to the island?' asks Steph.

'To be honest, I think I'm just really grateful bobbing along here,' I reply. 'I don't think there is enough daylight to get there and back comfortably and I don't want to disturb the birds. It is lovely to simply look at it from here.'

We turn back to the harbour, which was built in the late 1890s by the cove's benefactor at the time, Lord Robartes of Lanhydrock, to protect the pilchard fishing fleet from the wild Atlantic Ocean. While winter storms have always raged in this area, climate change means that the frequency and force of them has increased over the years, damaging the Grade-II-listed structure. The National Trust has made significant investments in repairing and maintaining the walls and thankfully they survived the power of the gales and waves of the 2014 winter storms.

As we paddle in, we can see people enjoying the sunset from the gardens of the Mullion Cove Hotel on the clifftop above. On the pier, wetsuit-clad girls and boys throw themselves with delight into the sea, scramble up the wall with the help of their friends and minutes later, launch themselves back in again,

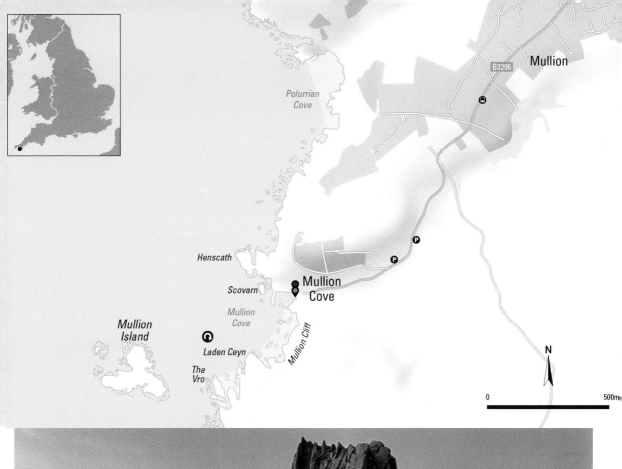

Mullion Island

Polurrian Cove

Henscath

Scovarn

Mullion Cove

Mullion Cove

Laden Ceyn

The Vro

Mullion Cliff

B3296

Mullion

N

0   500m

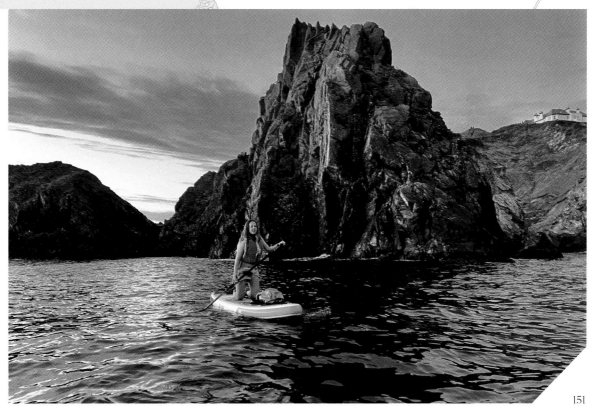

under the watchful eye of adults nearby. Picking up a plastic cup from the slip and tucking it into my buoyancy aid, I return to the car. We've barely covered any distance and have only been on the water for around 40 minutes, but the evening has been very special and has moved me deeply.

Looe and Mullion islands are reminders once again that as paddleboarders we are guests on the ocean, and there are, and should be, places we can only see from a distance.

Whether it is a resting seal or a nesting bird, what we do individually and collectively has an impact we need to be mindful of. I don't have the answers and I am not perfect, but I will continue to listen to and learn from the scientists and wardens whom know far more than me. I owe it to the marine and birdlife which call this home. I owe it too to the girls and boys on the harbour wall.

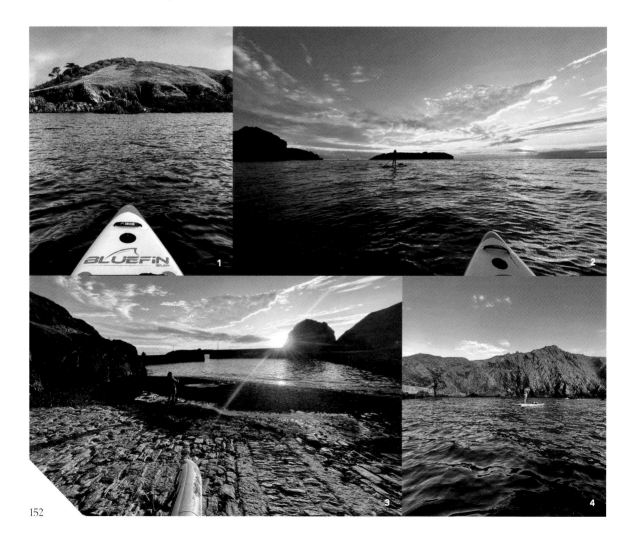

1 Looking towards Looe Island   2 The sunset at Mullion Island
3 Sunset at Mullion Cove   4 Dramatic cliffs near Mullion Cove

Technical information

DISTANCE
LOOE ISLAND **5.5km round trip.**
MULLION ISLAND **1.6km round trip.**
....
LAUNCH LOCATION
LOOE ISLAND
ENTRY AND EXIT POINT **SX 256523/50.345, -4.453**
TURN AROUND POINT **SX 258512/50.334, -4.449**
MULLION ISLAND
ENTRY AND EXIT POINT **SW 667179/50.015, -5.258**
TURN AROUND POINT **SW 663177/50.013, -5.263**
....
ALTERNATIVE ROUTES **Paddleboarding close
to Hannafore Beach would be lovely, as would
paddleboarding close to the harbour and along
the shore of Mullion Cove.**

Difficulty

Paddleboarding experience is necessary for
trips to both islands, and knowledge of wind
and tides is important.

Getting there

Looe Island

Looe Island is 1.5km from Looe in Cornwall.
Hannafore Beach is then just under 2km
from Looe.

There is a railway station in Looe, which has
connections to Liskeard. There is a bus from
Looe's railway station to Hannafore Point, which
carries on to Plymouth.

There is free parking along Marine Drive
by Hannafore Point (SX 256524/50.345, -4.453)
There are public toilets on the slope going to
the beach.

Mullion Island

The closest railway station is Redruth, with
connections to Plymouth, Cardiff and London.
A bus service from the station takes you to
Mullion, which is 28km away. From the bus stop
it is just over 1km to the launch point.

There is a car park around 500m from
the harbour run by Porthmellin Cafe
(SW 671180/50.017, -5.252). There is a larger
car park approximately 600m from the harbour
(SW 672181/50.018, -5.251). There are public
toilets on the way to the harbour.

Route information

The Hannafore Kiosk in Looe has a webcam,
and the Mullion Cove Hotel has one
overlooking Mullion Cove.

Eating and drinking

» The seasonal Island View Cafe serves
  salads, sandwiches, cakes and drinks.
  They also look after the
  #2MinuteBeachClean station.
» Hannafore Kiosk serves pasties, cakes,
  ice cream and hot drinks.
» Porthmellin Cafe in Mullion Cove serves
  cream teas, sandwiches and cakes.

Instruction, guided tours and equipment

» Adventure Fit Southwest runs guided tours
  and tuition.
» Vertical Blue Adventures offers mobile
  tuition, safaris and paddleboard hire.
» Lizard Adventure offers guided tours from
  Cadgwith Cove on the Lizard peninsula.

Further information

» Cornwall Wildlife Trust:
  www.cornwallwildlifetrust.org.uk
» Cornwall Seal Group Research Trust:
  www.cornwallsealgroup.co.uk
» Evelyn E Atkins, *We Bought an Island*
  (George G Harrap & Co Ltd, 1976)
  and *Tales From Our Cornish Island*
  (George G Harrap & Co Ltd, 1986).

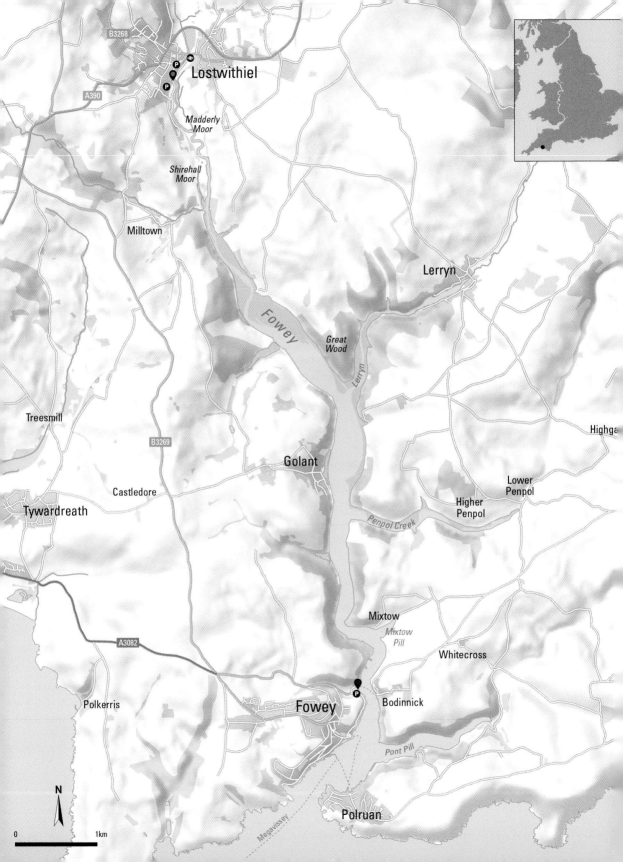

Lostwithiel

B3268

A390

Madderly Moor

Shirehall Moor

Milltown

Treesmill

B3269

Castledore

Tywardreath

Polkerris

A3082

Fowey

Golant

Great Wood

Lerryn

Lerryn

Penpol Creek

Higher Penpol

Lower Penpol

Highga

Mixtow

Mixtow Pill

Whitecross

Bodinnick

Pont Pill

Fowey

Mevagissey

Polruan

N

0   1km

Lostwithiel to Fowey Harbour, River Fowey

A TIDAL RIVER, *THE WIND IN THE WILLOWS*, SEASIDE BUNTING BLOWING IN THE BREEZE AND FUNDRAISING ADVENTURES

I'm in Fowey on a slightly overcast day with Steph Barnicoat, founder of SUP with Steph, who, with her trusty springer spaniel Percy, offers guided tours of The Gannel in Newquay in Cornwall. We're enjoying lunch overlooking the busy harbour and planning the next day's SUP adventure.

Steph is committed to sharing the benefits of paddleboarding for our mental well-being, and in the summer paddleboarded 96 kilometres along the Cornish coast fundraising for the mental health charity Mind Cornwall and Cal Major's Seaful. Day one of Steph's three-day challenge covered the journey I'm sharing with you today, a 19-kilometre paddle along the stunning River Fowey and estuary from Lostwithiel, passing Golant and then going on to Fowey Harbour where the estuary meets the English Channel.

The River Fowey rises at Fowey Well on Bodmin Moor on Cornwall's highest tor, Brown Willy, and winds its way for 43 kilometres to the sea. The valley from St Winnow is designated an Area of Outstanding Natural Beauty and the river runs through Golitha Falls, a National Nature Reserve rich in lichen, mosses and woodland flowers such as bluebells and wood anemone. The name Fowey comes from the river's Cornish name *Fowydh*, meaning beech trees, and the ancient woodland of Draynes Wood in Golitha Falls nature reserve was recorded in the Domesday Book in 1086.

Having parked my car in Fowey, we drive up to Lostwithiel, which lies at the head of the tidal section of the river, and launch close to high tide at a small slipway. It feels very special to be retracing the start of Steph's adventure, an idea she had dreamt of for some time before taking that first step to making it a reality. There are blue skies above as we paddle along a small channel passing the park and pretty sailing boats. The river gradually widens, twisting and turning as we move through the saltmarshes, and we spot swans, geese and ducks. Herons, kingfishers and egrets can be seen here too.

As clouds gather in the sky above, the river widens ahead of us, flanked by lush, green trees. To our left, close to the water's edge, is the church of St Winnow, where the churchyard is managed to promote biodiversity as a living churchyard. In the distance we spot Golant, a pretty village on our right, which would be a lovely launch spot for a shorter journey to Fowey. At low tide the exposed mudbanks and sandbars become feeding areas for wading birds.

We turn to our left and paddle a little way up Penpol Creek, exploring old wrecks and abandoned boats on the shore. I'd read about the wind picking up along the river and it certainly does as we fly along the creek before turning back and rejoining the river. A cormorant is drying its wings on one of the buoys and fishermen on their boats are chatting nearby as we paddle south. The beauty of the lower part of the estuary is believed to have been the inspiration for Kenneth Grahame's *The Wind in the Willows* after a boating trip he took here in 1907, as well as *Tales of the Riverbank*.

We are soon at Penmarlam Quay at Mixtow Pill and Fowey Docks, the latter of which Cornish China Clay is exported from. Ahead is Bodinnick, where the car ferry from Fowey lands and close to where we left my car. It is here at Ferryside that Daphne du Maurier, the author of *Rebecca*, *Frenchman's Creek* and *Jamaica Inn*

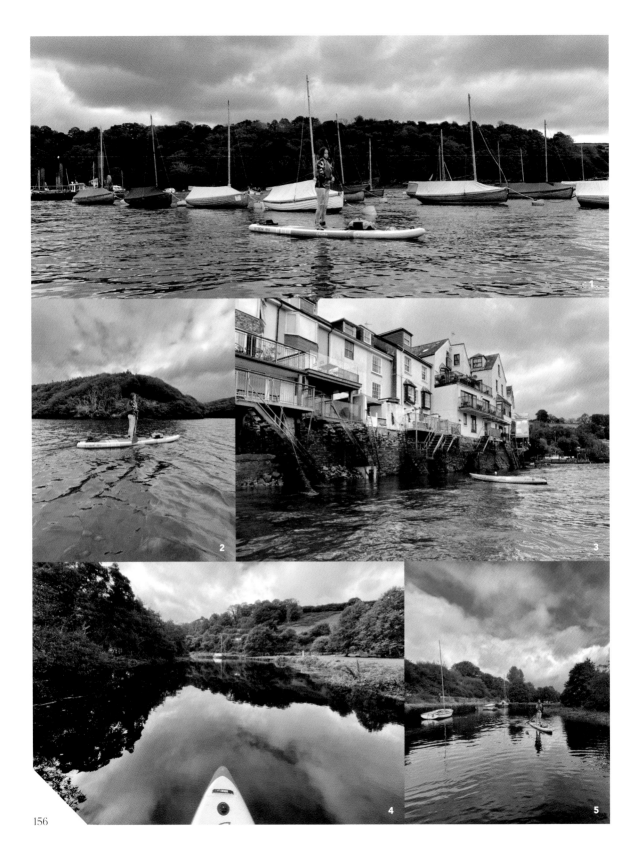

lived in the 1920s. The Fowey Festival of Arts and Literature is hosted each year by the Du Maurier Festival Society.

We are now in the harbour near Fowey's RNLI Trent-class, all-weather lifeboat, paddling along the quayside walls which, with the low tide, expose the harbour walls and ladders to the houses and steps into town. Once again paddling carefully around the boats and buoys as we did at Golant, we decide lunch can wait a little longer and make our way through slightly bigger waves to the mouth of the harbour, passing pastel-coloured homes and hotels above us.

Steph wants to show me St Catherine's Castle and the sheltered Readymoney Cove, which is cordoned off as a designated bathing beach. On the other side of the harbour is Polruan and as we return to the quayside we pass the ferry that runs between here and Fowey.

On her fundraising challenge, Steph would now have left the harbour to make her way westwards along the coast to Gweek. It has been a huge privilege to experience part of that route with her and I can only imagine the thrill she would have felt after months of planning.

It's most definitely time to eat and we leave the river by the Bodinnick ferry slipway, pack the boards away in my car and go in search of sandwiches and hot chocolate through the pretty streets of Fowey, bunting fluttering in the breeze and the buzz of late-summer holidaymakers enjoying the fresh air. We return to Lostwithiel together and say our goodbyes.

I take a quiet moment at the slipway where we launched, unaware of the beauty and sense of adventure that was about to unfold as the river and estuary revealed themselves. With careful planning and understanding of the wind and tides, this feels like a very special exploration of Cornwall's natural world. Even the dark clouds didn't dampen the joy.

1 Pretty sailing boats by Lostwithiel   **2** Steph paddling towards Golant   **3** The ladders up to Fowey
4 Perfectly still water   **5** Steph setting out from Lostwithiel

Technical information

DISTANCE **18km one way.**

LAUNCH LOCATION
ENTRY POINT **SX 104595/50.405, -4.669**
EXIT POINT **SX 127522/50.340, -4.634**

Difficulty

Paddleboarding experience is necessary for this trip and knowledge of wind and tides is important for the River Fowey if you're going independently. Launch at high tide at Lostwithiel or the mudbanks will be exposed.

Getting there

Lostwithiel

There is a railway station at Lostwithiel with connections to Plymouth, Bristol and Cardiff. Frequent buses to St Austell stop in Lostwithiel.

There is parking on Quay Street (SX 105597/50.406, -4.669) and also Coulson Park (SX 103593/50.404, -4.669). There are public toilets on Church Lane.

Fowey

The nearest railway stations to Fowey are Par and St Austell, both with connections to Plymouth, Bristol, London and Cardiff. There are bus routes from Par and St Austell to Fowey.

There is the pay-and-display Caffa Mill car park in Fowey (SX 126 522/50.340, -4.634), with paid public toilets.

Route information

In 2022, Fowey Harbour introduced a fee to paddleboard in the harbour: you must register your kit and pay £20 per year per board. Register at the harbour.

Please note, if you choose to launch in at Golant in front of the Fishermans Arms pub, be aware of the tide times and height. Over 5m and your car may get flooded.

Ferrymans Cottage holiday cottage has a webcam in Fowey.

Eating and drinking

» There are lots of places to eat in Fowey in the harbour, including Lazy Jacks Kitchen on Webb Street, which serves delicious sandwiches, ice cream and hot drinks.

Instruction, guided tours and equipment

» Paddle Cornwall SUP, based in Golant, offers tours and tuition.
» Fowey River Hire offers board hire and guided tours from Fowey.

Further information

» Fowey Festival of Arts and Literature: *www.foweyfestival.com*

Opposite The lush, green trees that greeted us as we set off

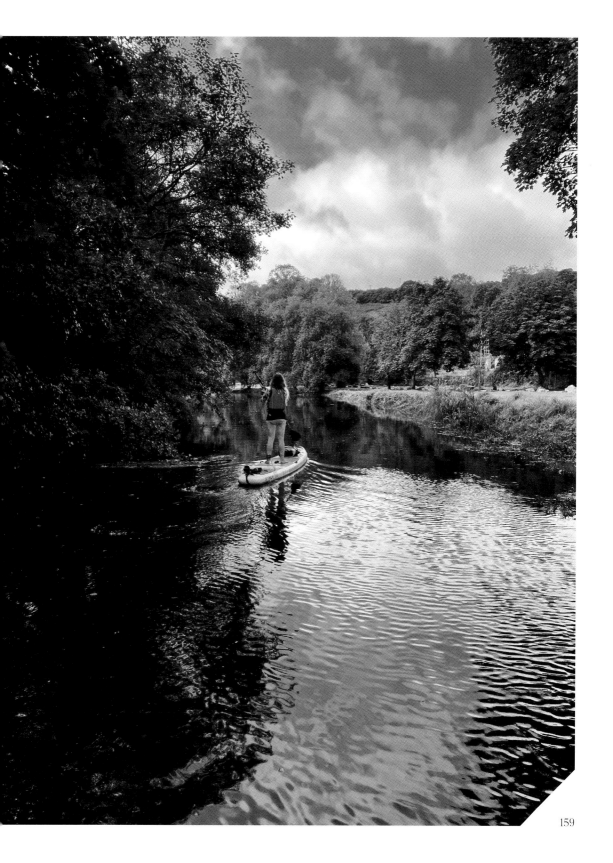

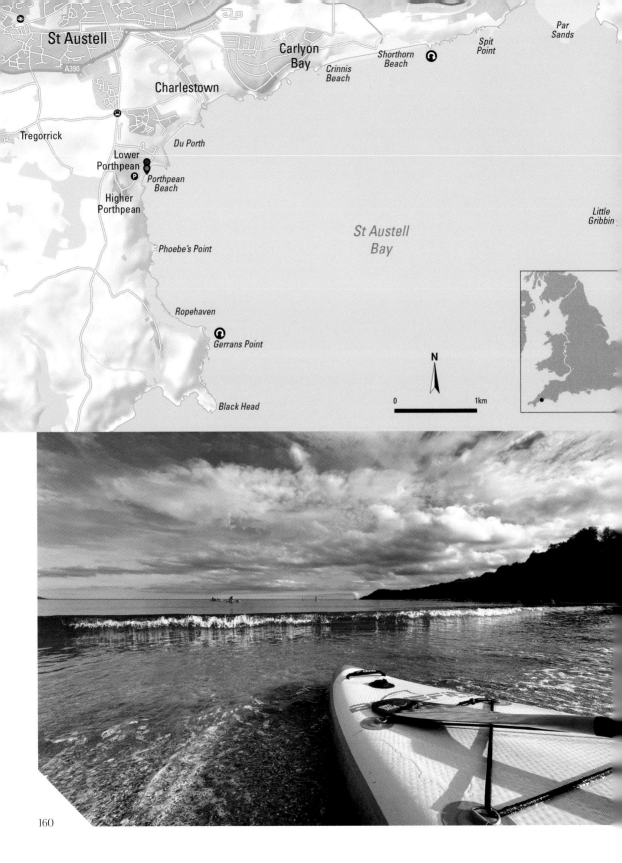

St Austell

Carlyon
Bay

Charlestown

Crinnis
Beach

Shorthorn
Beach

Spit
Point

Par
Sands

Tregorrick

Du Porth

Lower
Porthpean

Porthpean
Beach

Higher
Porthpean

Little
Gribbin

Phoebe's Point

St Austell
Bay

Ropehaven

Gerrans Point

Black Head

N

0   1km

Porthpean, St Austell

EXPLORING CAVES, GLITTER PATHS OF SUNLIGHT, PICNICS ON THE SEA AND A UNESCO WORLD HERITAGE SITE

'This is such a special place,' Steph says as we walk down the slip with our boards to Porthpean Beach. 'It is where I really understood what paddleboarding means to me. I also passed here on my way to Gweek on my fundraising challenge for Mind and Seaful. I really hope you like it.'

The early afternoon sun is shining as Steph Barnicoat – founder of SUP with Steph, adventurer and author – and I launch from a small, sheltered, sandy beach into St Austell Bay, along Cornwall's southern coastline, about five kilometres from St Austell. There are four brightly coloured kayaks lined up along the shore, families exploring the rock pools and a group of women dipping in the turquoise sea and laughing together. The water is warm, clear and calm as we paddle towards Black Head, a headland in the distance and the site of an Iron Age fort believed to be from the third century BC.

Steph wants to show me the caves, which we take a moment to explore. Everything is quiet but for the 'plop, plop' of copper-coloured water from the roof above. Beneath us the kelp sways gently, and rocks and sand are visible below. As we leave the cave, we meet three local kayakers and, unexpectedly, an inquisitive seal basking in the sunshine joins us momentarily before diving and swimming away.

The five of us paddle along, chatting together about our adventures for a few minutes. Hugging the coast, we pass three secluded beaches, accessed only from the sea, which are completely empty. How dreamy would it be to spend the day here, reading,

writing and enjoying a dip and a picnic?

Above is Ropehaven Cliffs Nature Reserve, owned by the Cornwall Wildlife Trust. The geology here is quite unusual for Cornwall, with thin, fossil-rich bands of limestone having been found. There are house martins and fulmars, a group of birds known as 'tubenoses' or 'petrels' that feed out at sea and return to the cliffs to nest in colonies on the high ledges. Running through the woodland is the South West Coast Path, which at 986 kilometres is one of the UK's longest national trails. It starts in Minehead in Somerset, follows the coastline of Cornwall, Devon and Dorset and finishes at Poole Harbour.

From Black Head we have a wonderful view of St Austell Bay and Steph points out the beaches we can see in the distance: Duporth, Charlestown, Carlyon Bay, Par, Polkerris and Menabilly, and round Gribbin Head to Fowey. As it's such a lovely afternoon, with blue skies and warm sunshine, she suggests we paddle across to Carlyon Bay, the caves and Charlestown, an eighteenth-century Georgian Harbour. I take the opportunity to ask Steph about her work in bioacoustics, tracking and studying how marine mammals such as whales use sound to navigate, search for food and avoid danger, as well as how human activity impacts their ability to do this successfully. I listen in wonder as we paddle along and she tells me about snorkelling with orcas in Norway.

Passing a mussel farm, we stop to chat to a paddleboarder that Steph knows from social media and for a few minutes, the three of us just bob on the sea talking about beautiful places to SUP in Cornwall.

An hour later we are at the other side of the bay and it's time for a picnic on our boards, our feet dangling in the warm seawater, before

Opposite Finishing our adventure at Porthpean Beach

we set off back to Porthpean. I can hear the sound of sails billowing in the wind and turn to see a beautiful boat with cream sheets and a black hull. It is the *Mascotte*, a Bristol Channel pilot cutter built in 1904 and thought to be the third-largest cutter of its type at 18.3 metres long, with a beam of 4.6 metres and twice as heavy as most others. Rich Clapham, originally from Oldbury on the River Severn, was her skipper for nine years and sailed her alongside the owner Mark Tyndall. In July 2019 Rich died by suicide. In his memory, Mark is setting up a new charitable trust called Rich's Boat. In their words:

'[The trust] hopes to provide opportunities for both total beginners and experienced sailors to push the boundaries of what they are capable of. It's all about sharing knowledge, skills and a positive life experience with those who may not otherwise have the opportunity to get out on the water or sail a boat as historically significant as *Mascotte*.'

She is moored in nearby Charlestown, a UNESCO World Heritage Site and working port built in the late 1700s that offers safe harbour for many traditional and historic sailing ships, as well as being a film location for programmes such as *Poldark*. Day trips on *Mascotte* and other sailing vessels such as *Anny of Charlestown* can be chartered here.

Our final stretch to Porthpean is a beautiful paddle following the glitter path of the late

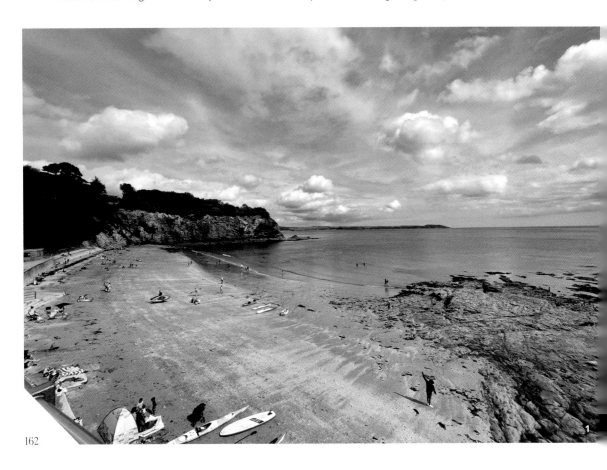

1 Porthpean Beach   **2** The cliffs of St Austell Bay   **3** Steph paddling as we make our way to Gerrans Point   **4** Looking back to Porthpean Beach

afternoon sun into a gentle breeze, lost in our thoughts but with the comforting companionship of a friend by our side, one of those moments so many paddleboarders cherish. As we return to Porthpean I notice an elegant white house set in the woods above. It looks familiar, although I can't place it. Perhaps an Agatha Christie mystery I love watching with my dad, I wonder?

What I do know is that Porthpean and St Austell Bay have been such interesting places to paddle which, in the right conditions, offer so much: caves to explore, big views, a long stretch of coastline, secluded beaches and historical Charlestown Harbour to paddle past. Choose a sunrise, sunset or daytime paddle and it will be different again. I can absolutely

understand why it is so special to Steph.

At my desk at home, I think back to the white house and discover it's not Poirot or Miss Marple, it's the location for *About Time*, a film with Bill Nighy about a young man, Tim, who has the ability to travel in time so that he can relive and change moments in the past. Watching the film again, Tim's words strike me: 'We're all travelling through time together, every day of our lives. All we can do is do our best to relish this remarkable ride.'

Porthpean and St Austell Bay offer a beautiful, remarkable ride on your paddleboard. I do hope you enjoy it as much as I did.

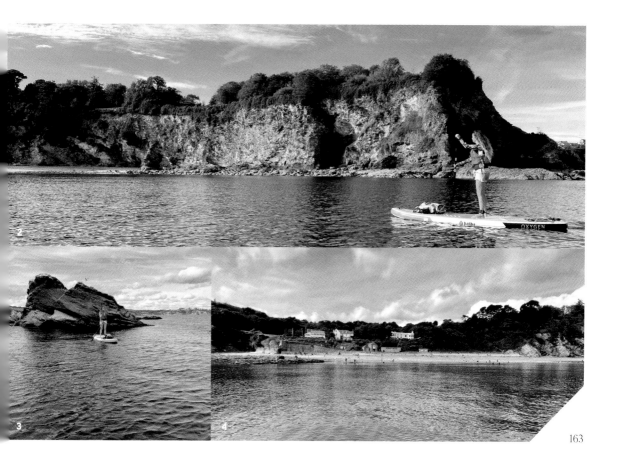

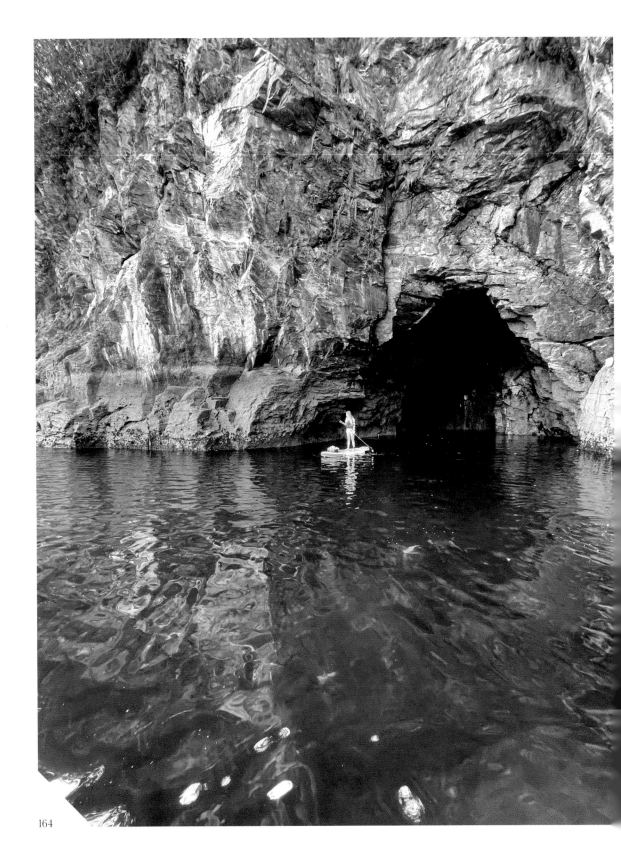

Technical information

DISTANCE **11km round trip.**

LAUNCH LOCATION
ENTRY AND EXIT POINT **SX 032 507/50.323, -4.766**
TURN AROUND POINT 1 **SX 041488/50.307, -4.751**
TURN AROUND POINT 2 **SX 067521/50.337, -4.717**

ALTERNATIVE ROUTE **Paddleboarding close to Porthpean Beach would be lovely.**

Difficulty

Paddleboarding experience is necessary for this trip and knowledge of wind and tides is important if you are going independently.

Getting there

Porthpean Beach is 4km from St Austell.

St Austell has a railway station with connections to Plymouth, Bristol, Cardiff and London. Buses from the railway station take you to Porthpean Road, just over a kilometre from Porthpean Beach. Buses to Fowey and Newquay also stop here.

There is a pay-and-display car park and seasonal toilets just by the beach (SX 031507/50.323, -4.768).

Route information

Porthpean Sailing Club has a webcam overlooking the beach.

Eating and drinking

» The seasonal Porthpean Beach Shop sells snacks and hot drinks.

Instruction, guided tours and equipment

» Cornwall Outdoors offers paddleboard hire. They are based at Porthpean Beach in the summer months.
» Amanda Leonard, founder of SUP in a Bag, offers tours in St Austell Bay, launching at Portmellon near Mevagissey.

Further information

» Rich's Boat: *www.richsboat.com*
» Charlestown Harbour: *www.charlestownharbour.com*

Opposite Exploring the caves near Porthpean Beach

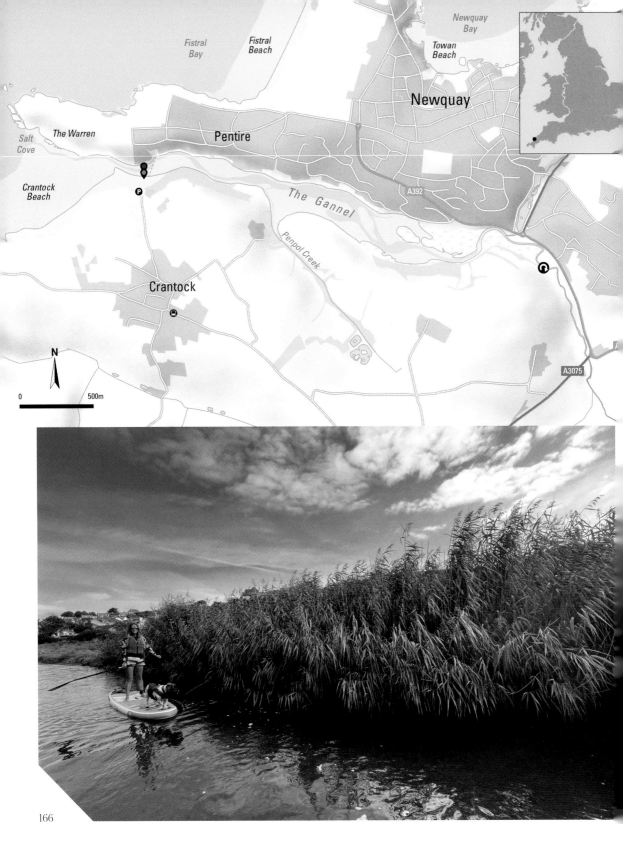

The Gannel, Newquay

DAWN STARTS, SUP WITH A PUP, LEARNING ABOUT SEALS AND THE RIVER'S WINDING CHANNEL

'So, I'm just checking the tides and wind for tomorrow,' she says, a mug of frothy hot chocolate in one hand, her phone in the other, 'and you need to be in Newquay for 7.15 a.m. for us to paddle The Gannel tomorrow.' I work backwards, adding half an hour for unexpected delays and my cautious driving. It's going to be a 5 a.m. start.

'Any wiggle room on the 7.15 a.m.?' I ask optimistically, biting into my tasty cheese-and-pickle sandwich from Lazy Jacks Kitchen.

With a twinkle in her eye, she says, 'Well, maybe 7.20 or 7.25 a.m. if you're really pushing it.'

I don't need the alarm to wake me the next day. Long before 'I Do Like to be Beside the Seaside' is set to ring on my phone, I am quietly tiptoeing out of my friend Louise's house and am on my way to Newquay, on Cornwall's north coast. As dawn breaks, my excitement grows, and even the smell of soggy kit can't dampen my spirits.

The dates for my Cornish research were built around the tide times of today's journey on the River Gannel a couple of months beforehand. This is how I discovered that Steph Barnicoat, aka SUP with Steph, was not only an adventurer and instructor but was also writing a book about beautiful places to SUP in Cornwall. Once again, I was struck by the generosity of the paddleboarding community when Steph offered to spend three days sharing wonderful locations with me – beaches, islands, caves, rivers, harbours and estuaries – all explored with picnics on our boards.

We have two special guests with us today: her springer spaniel Percy and Charlie, a Marine Stories Ranger with the award-winning marine conservation charity Cornwall Seal Group Research Trust. With a degree in Marine and Natural History Photography and a passion for the ocean as a diver and paddleboarder, Charlie is the perfect person to share the unique stories of seals and how we can protect them. I have so many questions to ask her, and where better to talk than on a SUP?

The National Trust car park by Crantock Beach is already filling up when we arrive and begin pumping our boards. I run to the top of the sand dunes and look out at the beach where the River Gannel spills into the Celtic Sea. To my left there are surfers in the waves and dog walkers under blue skies, white, fluffy clouds and a gentle breeze. We walk past the Big Green Surf School and launch on to The Gannel in the sunshine, the tide still coming in and the water warm and clear. It is everything I had secretly hoped for and more.

The River Gannel rises on Newlyn Downs, an area designated a Site of Special Scientific Interest, and journeys west for 11 kilometres, dividing the town of Newquay on the south side from Crantock village. The Gannel estuary, where the freshwater river meets the ocean, is an important habitat for wading birds, and Steph sees egrets and sometimes herons too. We paddle past ducks and are lucky enough to later spy a pristine great white egret in the distance.

The area has a long tradition as a trading site, with Celtic and Roman coins being found in the fields along the estuary. As we head upstream, to our right is Penpol Creek, where cargo was transported inland by cart or packhorse. At low tide you can see the mooring rings, steps, chains and quays from these times. Up until the nineteenth century, The Gannel

Opposite The reeds of The Gannel estuary

was also used for shipping goods that arrived at Fern Pit on the opposite bank. Schooners and flat-bottomed barges, known as lighters, would then be poled or rowed up the river to Trevemper, carrying timber, coal and sand to inland mining and agricultural industries. Today it is the Fern Pit Cafe & Ferry, a family-run business established in 1910, that carries visitors on the ferry boat *Sunshine* from the East Pentire headland across the river to Crantock Beach when the tide is in. When the tide is out, there is a footbridge across the estuary which we can just about see through the water below.

A group of women are laughing as they enjoy a morning swim by the bank and a family splash joyfully on their paddleboard. There are small sailing boats and walkers pausing for a cup of tea at the picnic table on the path.

As we paddle leisurely in the sunshine, I chat to Charlie about the Cornwall Seal Group Research Trust and how as paddleboarders we can ensure that we behave responsibly while enjoying the chance to share the sea with these incredible marine mammals. She explains that seals – especially pregnant females, pups, juveniles under a year and the dominant 'beachmaster' males – are most vulnerable when when they are hauled out on a beach or rocks. If we disturb them by getting too close, there is the risk the seals will stampede (rush into the sea) or tombstone (throw themselves from a height above the water line). This is always a waste of energy, often leads to injury and can be fatal. In the wild every calorie counts and can make the difference between life and death. It's therefore important that we keep at least 100 metres away from any hauled-out seal.

If we see a seal in the water, again the key is to keep a distance, stay quiet and, if we can, keep downwind so they can't smell us. Splashing their flippers or making a noise is a sign of distress, indicating that we are too close and they feel threatened. If a seal comes close to our boards, as the pup did to mine in Cullercoats (p83), then it is usually simply being inquisitive and is approaching on its own terms. If a seal follows you, again because it is curious, keep moving – it will lose interest if you don't engage with it.

By now, the tide has turned and the water is getting shallower as we make our way to the marshy area and reeds through the river channels, spotting the pretty pink and yellow, daisy-like sea aster. It is this sense of discovery as we begin to see what the receding tide reveals that I find so interesting about an estuary. On the highest spring tide, The Gannel could be over seven metres deep. Now, as we return to the launch point the river's channel winding through the sandbanks is so much clearer.

The beach is now busier, with dogs playing in the sea, RNLI flags showing where it is safe to swim, queues for ice cream and cake at Cargo Coffee and lots of easy weekend relaxing in deckchairs. On a slightly longer walk back to the car, we chat to Steph's friends at the Big Green Surf School and load up the boards on the roof rack.

Our morning together has been everything I had hoped for all those weeks ago: paddling, learning how we can protect the seals around the coastline, watching Percy enjoying the sunshine and exploring the everchanging Gannel. A very early start and slightly soggy kit were most definitely worth it.

1 Crantock Beach   **2** Percy enjoying his paddle

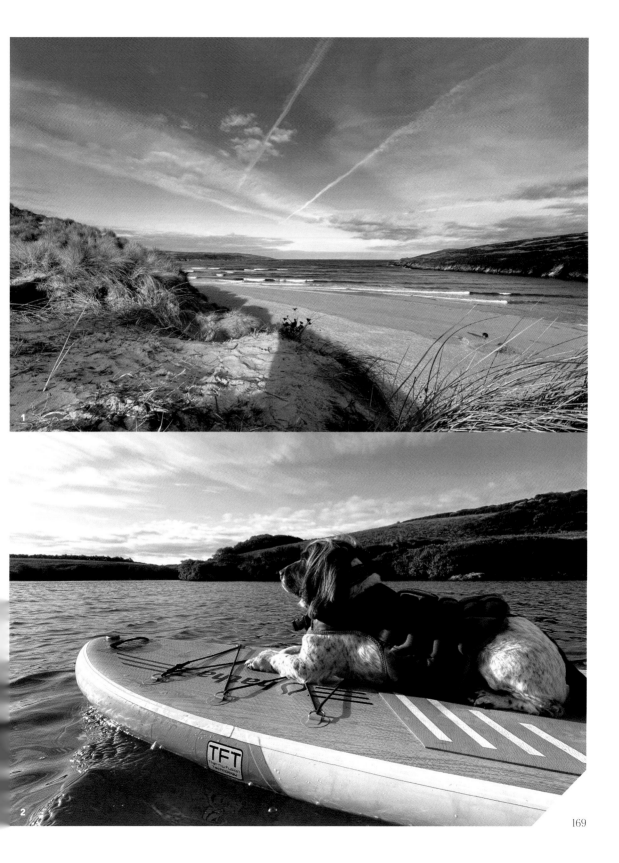

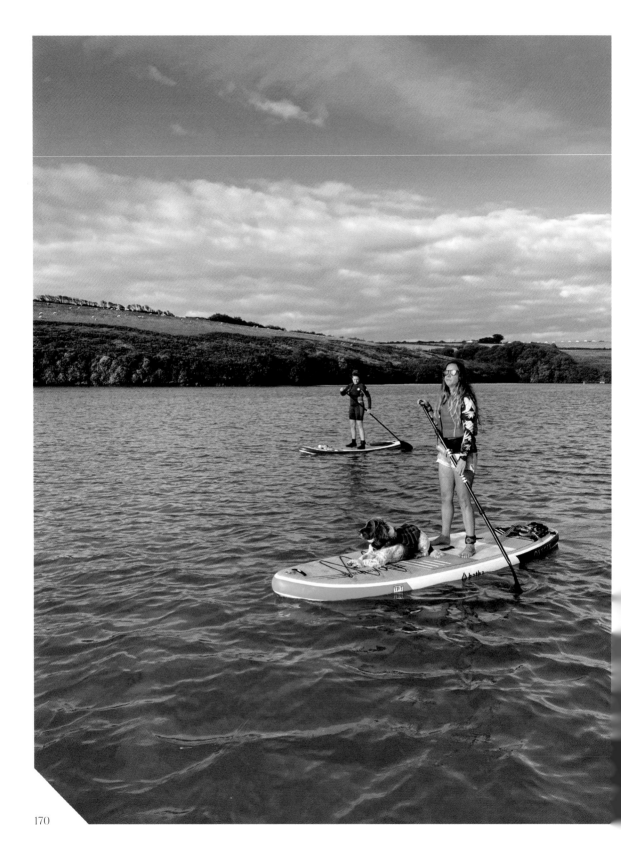

Technical information

DISTANCE **7.5km round trip.**

LAUNCH LOCATION
ENTRY AND EXIT POINT **SW 789611/50.408, -5.112**
TURN AROUND POINT **SW 816605/50.404, -5.075**

Difficulty

Paddleboarding experience is necessary for a trip along The Gannel and knowledge of wind and tides is important if you're going independently.

When the water height is lower than 6m the water is very shallow in some areas, making it annoying for large fins – it will be fine if you can keep in the river channel. The Gannel should be avoided if there are strong easterly/westerly winds as it funnels through. In other directions you can find shelter.

Getting there

The Gannel and Crantock Beach where we launched are about 4km from Newquay.

You can reach Newquay by rail from Par. There is a bus to Crantock village from Newquay railway station. There is then a walk of around 700m to the beach.

The pay-and-display car park at Crantock Beach is owned by the National Trust (SW 788610/50.407, -5.113) – members of the National Trust can park for free. There is a 2.1m height barrier which is opened 9 a.m. to 5 p.m., April to October only. There are toilets in the car park.

Route information

There are RNLI lifeguards on Crantock Beach during the summer months.

The Bowgie Inn pub and Crantock Bay holiday apartments each have a webcam over Crantock Beach.

Eating and drinking

» Cargo Coffee on Crantock Beach sells sandwiches, drinks and ice cream.

Instruction, guided tours and equipment

» Steph Barnicoat, who runs SUP with Steph in Newquay, offers guided tours and instruction on The Gannel.
» Big Green Surf School is based at Crantock Beach car park and offers guided tours, board hire and instruction.
» Newquay Activity Centre offers SUP lessons and tours, snorkel and SUP adventures and SUP and bushcraft tours.

Further information

» Cornwall Seal Group Research Trust: *www.cornwallsealgroup.co.uk*

Opposite A joyful paddle with Steph, Percy and Charlie

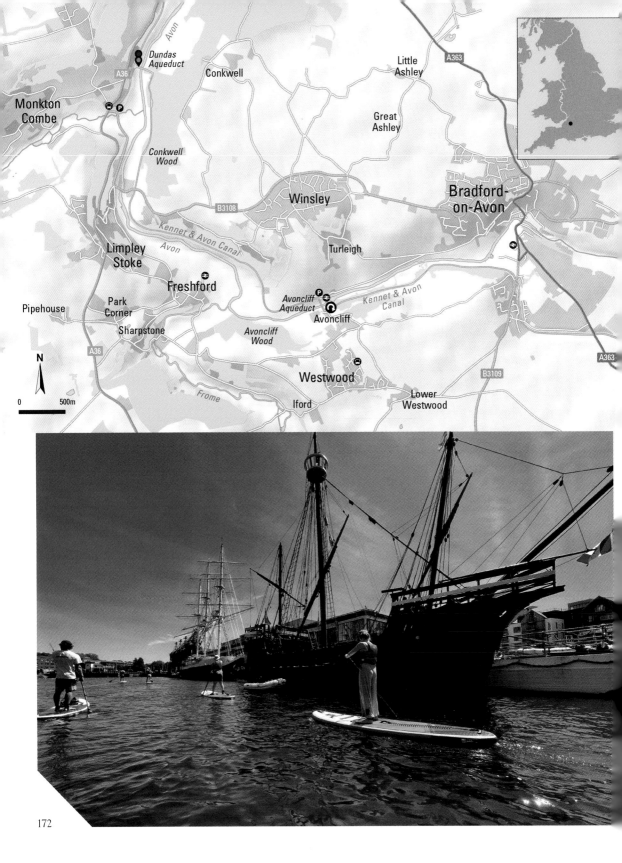

Dundas
Aqueduct

Conkwell

Little
Ashley

A363

Monkton
Combe

A36

Great
Ashley

Conkwell
Wood

Winsley

Bradford-
on-Avon

B3108

Kennet & Avon Canal

Limpley
Stoke

Avon

Turleigh

Freshford

Avoncliff
Aqueduct

Kennet & Avon
Canal

Pipehouse

Park
Corner

Avoncliff

Sharpstone

Avoncliff
Wood

A36

Westwood

A363

B3109

N

Frome

Iford

Lower
Westwood

0   500m

Bristol Harbourside and Kennet and Avon Canal

SS *GREAT BRITAIN*, A VIBRANT HARBOUR, BUTTERFLIES AND A HISTORIC AQUEDUCT

Possibilities and inspiration – these are the two words that spring to mind when I think of Bristol. Over the last few years I have been fortunate enough to attend the Women's Adventure Expo and Shextreme Film Festival in Bristol. It was there I first heard world-record paddleboarder, ocean advocate and founder of Seaful, Cal Major, speak so passionately about how as paddleboarders we have the opportunity to look after the oceans and inland waterways. I remember walking around the harbour, exploring the history of the Underfall Yard, looking up at Hotwells and the beautiful, brightly coloured homes on the skyline and wondering if one day I would be brave enough to fulfil my own SUP dream.

Only a year before I had been told that my idea to paddle coast to coast across Northern England was logistically too complex and physically too difficult for a woman of my age. Unsure of myself, I had tucked the dream away. 'Their courage to follow their passions and the "whispers in their heart" inspires me to continue to work on mine,' I wrote in my journal in 2017 as I boarded the train home. A year later, I would meet Frit Tam of Passion Fruit Pictures in Bristol and we would go on to become firm friends as I paddled from Liverpool to Goole and create our film *Brave Enough – A Journey Home to Joy*. Therefore, the opportunity to experience both the buzz of the city that had inspired me so much and the gentler Kennet and Avon Canal near Bath, with the award-winning SUP Bristol founded by Tim Trew and Kate Ingham, was something I knew

would be very special.

The Kennet and Avon Canal is a 140-kilometre-long canal linking London with the Bristol Channel. Made up of three historic waterways (the Kennet Navigation, the Avon Navigation and the Kennet and Avon Canal) and with 104 locks, it was completed in 1810. However, it struggled to compete with the Great Western Railway which opened in 1841. The canal continued to decline and in the 1960s fell into disrepair. A group of waterways enthusiasts and locals formed the Kennet and Avon Canal Trust and brought the canal back to life. I'm so grateful they did.

It is already a hot and sunny morning when Jamie from SUP Bristol, a group of friends and I launch at Brassknocker Basin near Monkton Combe and cross the beautiful Dundas Aqueduct. As we paddle along the 137-metre-long aqueduct, cyclists, runners, walkers and canoeists are all enjoying this flourishing spot. Carrying the canal over the River Avon, it is so important historically that it was the first canal structure to be designated a Scheduled Ancient Monument, which, according to the Canal & River Trust, makes it as important as Stonehenge.

Lined with overhanging trees, reeds and yellow flag iris, the canal offers paddleboarders a lovely, winding journey through lush countryside. Butterflies, ducklings, damselflies and dragonflies join us as we make our way to Avoncliff Aqueduct, about five kilometres away. The soft, honey-coloured stone bridges and homes look gorgeous, along with old wooden moorings that double as help for the ducks to reach the towpath.

Opposite A view many visitors won't experience

At Avoncliff, a pretty village lying within the Cotswolds Area of Outstanding Natural Beauty, we paddle across the 100-metre aqueduct and then stop to pull our boards out of the water. Time for a picnic lunch in the sun by the River Avon, close by the Cross Guns Avoncliff pub. We had planned to SUP the river back to our launch point, however as it offers little shade we return along the canal. One for a cooler day …

Arriving back at Brassknocker Basin and the small stretch of the Somerset Coal Canal, I look up at the majestic trees on the hill. I spot a narrowboat, the Dawdling Dairy, on the aqueduct selling ice cream. What could be more perfect after a sunny day's paddling on the Kennet and Avon Canal, I wonder?

The next morning, the sun shines brightly as we launch from the slipway at Baltic Wharf near the Harbour Masters Office and The Cottage Inn pub on Bristol's harbour. A pair of swans pass nonchalantly as we head towards the Bristol Marina, the SS *Great Britain* and the Floating Harbour. The SS *Great Britain* (SS meaning steam ship) was designed by Victorian engineer Isambard Kingdom Brunel and launched on 19 July 1843 from Bristol. She was the largest ship in the world at the time and the first to be built from wrought iron with a screw propeller. Her flags flutter in the wind and she looks majestic as we paddle past and enjoy a view most visitors to the museum won't experience.

The harbourside is buzzing as people go about their day: runners and cyclists whizz by, families walk together and friends chat at the cafes. How wonderful for the paddleboarders of Bristol to see familiar places from a new perspective and to have this blue adventure in the heart of their city. To my right on Prince's Wharf I see the M Shed, where I had heard Cal Major speak, and to my left the Arnolfini where the film festival had inspired me. 'Thank you,' I quietly say to myself.

As we reached Prince Street Bridge we turn round, heading back to the slipway and the promise of a cup of tea and delicious flapjack at the Underfall Cafe. The breeze has strengthened and paddling into the wind I pass, quite unintentionally, one of my fellow paddlers. 'Have you put an engine on your board?' she jokes.

'Ha, ha!' I reply. 'No, I just think I really love Bristol Harbour!'

Passing the Lloyds Amphitheatre and the iconic brightly coloured homes on our right, I once again feel the courage and excitement I had written about in 2017. There's something special about Bristol that never fails to make me feel braver.

With a full heart and spring in my step, I board the bus for a long journey home, reflecting once again upon the possibilities and inspiration Bristol and Bath offer. The contrast of the gentle Kennet and Avon Canal with the vibrancy of Bristol Harbourside make the experience of each even more special than I had anticipated. I do hope you will have the opportunity to enjoy both.

Opposite Aprroaching a stone bridge on the Kennet and Avon Canal

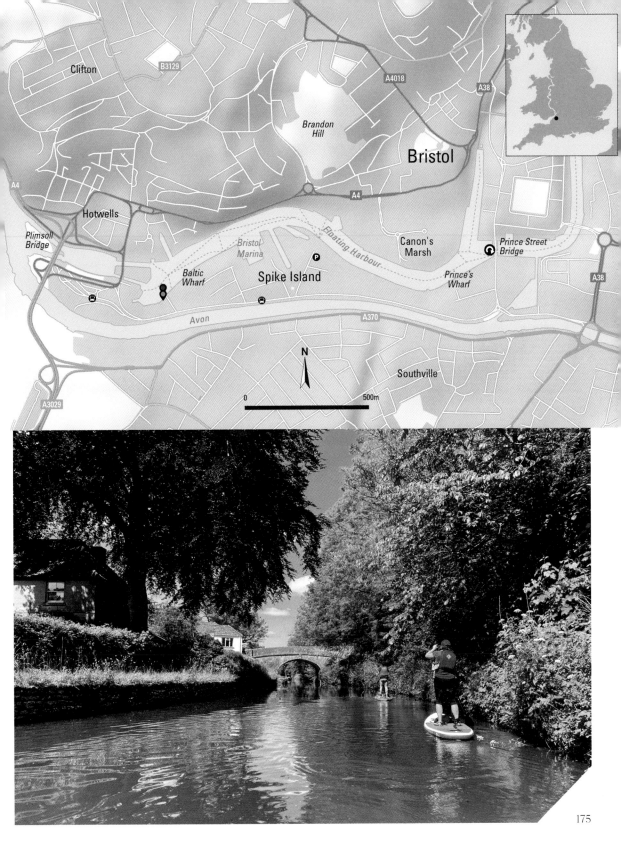

Technical information

DISTANCE
KENNET AND AVON CANAL **10km round trip.**
BRISTOL HARBOURSIDE **5km round trip.**
....
LAUNCH LOCATION
KENNET AND AVON CANAL
ENTRY AND EXIT POINT **ST 784625/51.361, -2.312**
TURN AROUND POINT **ST 805600/51.339, -2.283**
BRISTOL HARBOURSIDE
ENTRY AND EXIT POINT **ST 573722/51.447, -2.617**
TURN AROUND POINT **ST 586723/51.448, -2.597**

Difficulty

Kennet and Avon Canal

Canals are usually flat and a good place to build your confidence and technical skills. Be aware of narrowboats and other canal users. There are no locks on this stretch.

Bristol Harbourside

This is a lovely place to build your confidence and technical skills. Be aware of other boat users. Friends who paddle in Bristol regularly say the wind can pick up throughout the day, so the morning is best if possible. Be aware of others using the water, for example rowing clubs.

Getting there

Kennet and Avon Canal

To get to Brassknocker Basin, there are buses from Bath city centre and Salisbury which stop just by the launch point.

For Avoncliff Aqueduct, there are buses to Bath city centre and Bradford-on-Avon which stop in Westwood, just over 1km from the aqueduct.

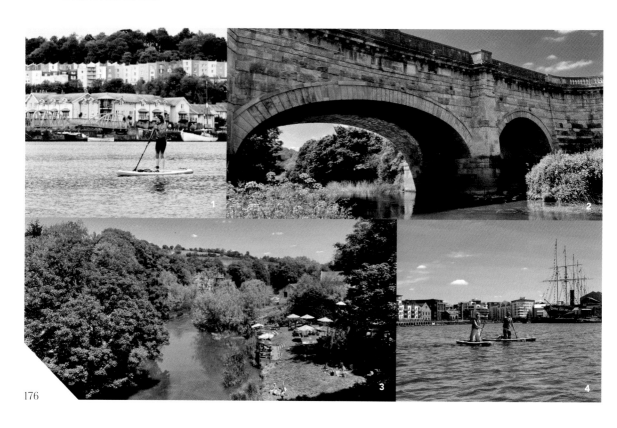

Avoncliff railway station is next to the aqueduct and has connections to Bath, Bristol, Bradford-on-Avon and Trowbridge. You must be in a specific carriage to alight at Avoncliff. Why not use the railway and paddle this route with a launch and exit point at Avoncliff?

A pay and display at Brassknocker Basin is run by the Somerset Coal Canal Society (ST 782621/51.358, -2.314).

There is a small, privately owned pay-and-display car park at Avoncliff (ST 804601/51.340, -2.282).

Bristol Harbourside

Bristol is widely connected by rail, bus and car. I took the National Express and walked to the harbour, which is a walk of about 2.5km.

Bristol Temple Meads railway station is about 3km from the harbour and has connections throughout Britain, including Portsmouth, Cardiff, Newcastle, London and Edinburgh. Buses throughout Bristol are available 500m east from the launch point. The Visit Bristol website has information on local buses and FirstGroup buses run near the harbourside.

There is a pay and display at the Maritime Heritage Centre short-stay car park (ST 579723/51.448, -2.607).

Route information

If you wish to use your own paddleboard and SUP independently in Bristol Harbourside, you will need to apply for a manually propelled vessels licence, launch from the slipway, wear a life jacket or buoyancy aid and take note of the Underfall Yard area exclusion zone. You can apply for a day licence for one day only (approximately £8 in 2022) or an annual licence that runs from May to April (approximately £40

in 2022). To apply for a day licence, you need to visit the Harbour Masters Office on the day in person. Phone 01179 031484 or email *harbour.office@bristol.gov.uk* for more information. You can apply for an annual licence online at *www.bristol.gov.uk*

If you are a member of British Canoeing, the insurance that comes with that covers you. If not, insurance will be added to your licence for an extra fee.

A Waterways Licence is required for the Kennet and Avon Canal.

Eating and drinking

» The Angelfish Restaurant at Brassknocker Basin.
» The Dawdling Dairy ice cream narrowboat sits on Brassknocker Basin.
» At the Cross Guns Avoncliff there is also Darcy Pies deli serving baguettes, cakes, smoothies, ice cream and, of course, pies at limited times throughout the year in the garden of the pub.
» Underfall Cafe is a short walk from the launch point at Bristol Harbourside. The flapjack, tea and warm welcome were perfect. They also do breakfast baps and lunchtime sandwiches.
» The Cottage Inn pub on the harbourside in Bristol.

Instruction, guided tours and equipment hire

» This is a route for those who have their own boards. Alternatively, book a guided tour with the SUP Bristol team. I paddled with SUP Bristol in the harbour and used their board. They also offer courses to improve your skills, guided tours in the UK and abroad.

1 The pretty houses on the edge of Bristol Harbour © Red Paddle Co/SUP Bristol **2** The River Avon from the Avoncliff Aqueduct **3** The lush River Avon **4** Bristol Harbour, with the SS *Great Britain* in the distance

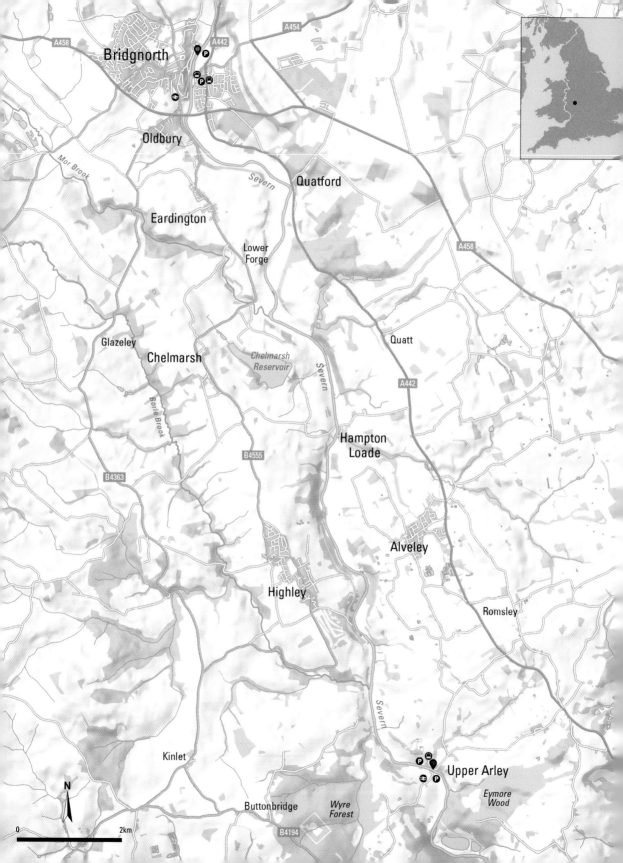

Bridgnorth

A458

A442

A454

Oldbury

Mor Brook

Severn

Quatford

Eardington

A458

Lower
Forge

Glazeley

Chelmarsh

Chelmarsh
Reservoir

Quatt

Borle Brook

Severn

A442

Hampton
Loade

B4555

Alveley

B4363

Highley

Romsley

Kinlet

Severn

Upper Arley

Eymore
Wood

N

Buttonbridge

Wyre
Forest

0   2km

B4194

Bridgnorth, River Severn

SPOTTING KINGFISHERS AND OTTERS, LEARNING THE LANGUAGE OF RIVERS AND A HERITAGE STEAM RAILWAY

One of the joys of paddleboarding is that we can learn to paddle in a relatively short time, and yet there is always a new body of water to explore, learn about and build our technical skills on. When Craig Jackson, Operational Fire Officer for Shropshire Fire and Rescue Service, SUP river guide and coach, ambassador for Seaful, father to lovely Edward and husband to Emily, invited me to paddle the River Severn with him, I knew it would be a perfect chance to visit somewhere beautiful and understand more about the wonders and lessons of paddleboarding on rivers.

I have some river experience – a magical summer evening on the River Dee, two glorious days on the River Aire through Leeds and on to the beautiful RSPB Fairburn Ings Nature Reserve, as well as a short river section in the Lake District back in 2016 during my first lesson. However, on that occasion, like many beginners, I was more worried about not falling in and have scant memory of flow or features.

As we paddle through Shrewsbury at dusk, Craig reminds me of the rules of the river ahead of our longer adventure on the River Severn the next day. 'If you're on your board looking downstream, then the left-hand bank is river left. If you're looking upstream, although the same bank will now be on your right it is still referred to as river left,' he explains. 'It'll be helpful to know so we can alert each other to anglers or eddies by the riverbank tomorrow.'

I have been reading Tristan Gooley's *How to Read Water* and fall asleep with my head buzzing with Craig's tips on eddies, scribbling notes in the margin.

The River Severn is the longest river in Britain at 354 kilometres long, rising near the River Wye in the Cambrian Mountains and finally reaching the sea in the Bristol Channel. It flows through Shrewsbury, Worcester and Gloucester. You may perhaps have heard of the famous Severn Bore? The bore is created because the river has a very high tidal range – the highest in the UK – and due to the shape of the estuary, water on an incoming tide is funneled into a narrowing channel. As the tide rises a large wave travelling against the river's current forms, which experienced surfers and SUP surfers can ride. According to William Thomson in his excellent book *The Book of Tides*, Colonel Jack Churchill, a World War Two veteran who had been awarded a medal for bravery and was known affectionately as 'Mad Jack', became the first person in the world to surf a tidal bore. The record for the longest surf is over an hour.

We absolutely aren't SUP surfing the River Severn, but Craig does have an exciting adventure planned, with a final surprise twist. We (Craig and his friends Alex and Chloe) launch from the slip by the playground in Severn Park, Bridgnorth. We have a 17-kilometre paddle ahead, and Arley station is our destination. Paddling downstream, we will leave the river, deflate our boards and return to Bridgnorth on the heritage Severn Valley Railway.

We drop to our knees for more stability as we pass under a bridge and over shallow rocks, and are on our way. Trees line the riverbank, gradually rising high above us on the hills. Perched on their branches, the birds are singing. Ducks, geese and swans pass by. The flow of the river gently carries us along. Then, ahead of us, Alex spots the unmistakable

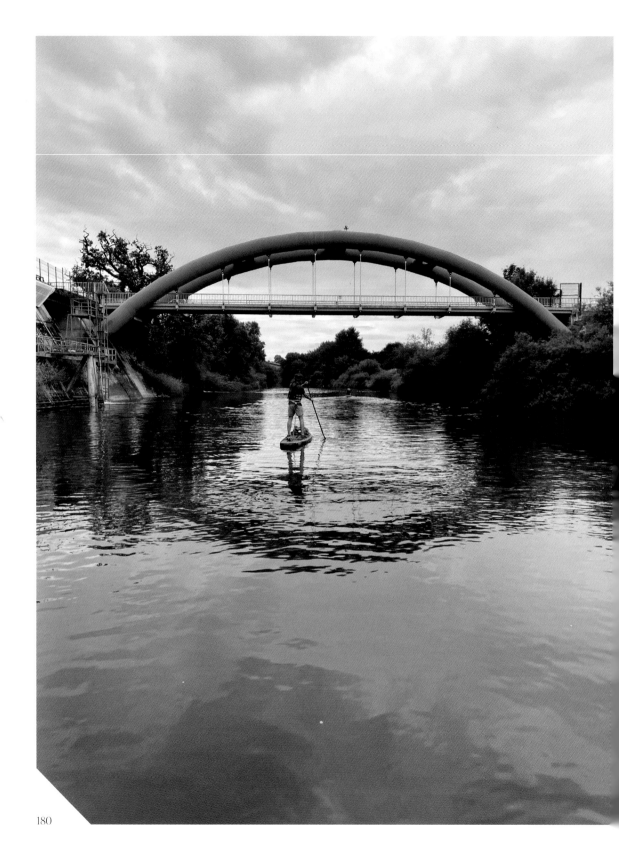

electric blue of a kingfisher in flight. Five years of paddleboarding and this is my first kingfisher – what beauty!

As the river bends to the right a cliff of red sandstone stands proudly above us. Another bend and we spy a gorgeous cottage set back from the bank. Add a sprinkling of snow and a steaming mug of hot chocolate and we could be in a feel-good Christmas film. Every so often we kneel to add stability and ride across the small rapids. I start to see the different patterns of water across the rocks and my confidence and excitement grows. We paddle along, soaking up the chance to be in the fresh air together, asking about each other's paddleboarding adventures and what it means to us. I'm always struck by how quickly a shared joy for paddleboarding opens up conversations that everyday life simply doesn't allow for.

Passing more homes on the left, we spot the entrance to a tunnel and can hear the sound of water gushing. Eager to explore more, after leaving our boards on the bank we peek through the running water to a beautiful waterfall. It feels magical: the river is sharing hidden treasures. There is a small island ahead with the water flowing more rapidly over the rocks on the left, and we decide to stop for our picnic in the sunshine to our right. Tucking into brownies, we see Alex, who is also a SUP instructor, waving and mouthing 'otter'. For 10 minutes we all stand quietly watching the river in the hope it may appear again. It doesn't, but we are thrilled Alex has seen it. How often, I wonder, do adults pause to simply watch for wildlife?

The huffing and hissing of the Severn Valley heritage steam train gets louder, and from the river we can see it pass through the trees.

'We better get a move on,' calls Craig, 'we have a train to catch!'

After carrying our boards across a shallow, rocky outcrop, we pick up speed passing through the Severn Valley Country Park, 126 acres of stunning countryside. A photographer is patiently watching for sand martins on the bank and an inquisitive duck is enjoying the contents of an angler's lunch box nearby.

At Arley we stop at the slipway to pack up our belongings and walk five minutes up the hill to the station, where *The Explorer* is set to arrive. A beautiful steam train pulls in and the guard allows us to stow our bags in an empty luggage carriage while we find our seats. Sun-kissed, relaxed and happily tired, we chat, finish off the flapjack and look down upon the river we have just paddled.

Leaving the train at Bridgnorth, Craig has one more surprise in store as we cross the bridge and make our way back to Severn Park: a ride in the oldest and steepest inland electric funicular railway in England, Bridgnorth Cliff Railway. As we descend the 34-metre-high sandstone cliffs on the Bridgnorth Cliff Railway, I can't help but smile.

Rivers like the Severn do require thought and planning, but they are so worth it. A kingfisher, otter, rapids and now two special railway rides, the River Severn has been a magical SUP adventure. I hope you'll experience that magic too.

Opposite Paddleboarding near South Staffs Water at Hampton Loade

Technical information

DISTANCE **17km one way.**

LAUNCH LOCATION
ENTRY POINT **SO 720934/52.538, -2.414**
EXIT POINT **SO 765801/52.418, -2.346**

ALTERNATIVE ROUTE **Instead of taking the steam railway back, you could park one car at Arley and do a shuttle trip if you are paddling with friends, or alternatively book a taxi.**

Difficulty

Paddleboarding on rivers takes planning, thought and an understanding of the obstacles and the equipment required.

Getting there

The heritage Bridgnorth railway station, which has refreshments and toilets, is just over 1km from the launch point, with connections to Kidderminster. The nearest mainline station is Wolverhampton, with connections across Britain including London, Edinburgh, Aberystwyth, Birmingham and Manchester. From the railway station you can then get a bus to Bridgnorth, which will take you within 300m of the launch location. National Express services across Britain from Wolverhampton are also available.

There is a pay-and-display car park in Severn Park (SO 721934/52.538, -2.412). We launched from the slipway near here.

From the exit point, Arley's heritage railway is just a few hundred metres away. Buses to Kidderminster can be caught 500m north of the exit point.

At the exit point, there are car parks on both the north (SO 762803/52.420, -2.351) and south (SO 766800/52.418, -2.346) of the river.

Route information

Please note that a Waterways Licence is required from Stourport-on-Severn to Gloucester. The section from Pool Quay near Welshpool and Stourport does not require a licence. The section below Gloucester is tidal and therefore does not require a licence.

Also, while the stream that gushed like a

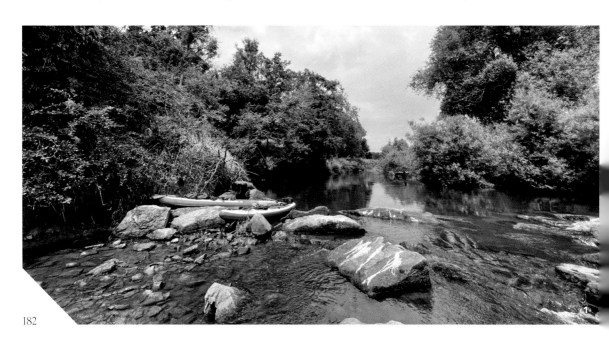

1 Our lunch spot   **2** Chloe, Alex and Craig paddling   **3** Bridgnorth Cliff Railway

waterfall was clean when when we were there, it does have an outlet further away that could discharge sewage at times of heavy rain or flooding. Craig and I researched this on the Rivers Trust website and found that in 2020 the sewer overflowed and spilled twice for a total of an hour. For 90 per cent of the year it would be clean water, however this raises an important question about the challenges we face regarding river pollution.

Ensure that if you stop for lunch on your journey that you do so on a public access point. Where this isn't possible then spots on the river where the riverbed is exposed, such as islands or beaches, are advised, but be aware that you may still be trespassing. Always be considerate to landowners and their livestock.

Eating and drinking

» We took our own picnics, but the Arley Riverside Tea Rooms in Upper Arley looked lovely.

Instructions, guided tours and equipment hire

» Craig Jackson runs guided tours of the River Severn at SUP Shropshire Adventure Guiding.
» Alex Chester runs SUP Shrewsbury, where you can take lessons, guided tours and hire boards.

Further information

» Seaful: *www.seaful.org.uk*
» The Rivers Trust: *www.theriverstrust.org*
» Severn Valley Railway: we travelled on the heritage steam railway from Arley station to Bridgnorth. There are toilets at Arley station and a cafe open at weekends: *www.svr.co.uk*
» Bridgnorth Cliff Railway: *www.bridgnorthcliffrailway.co.uk*

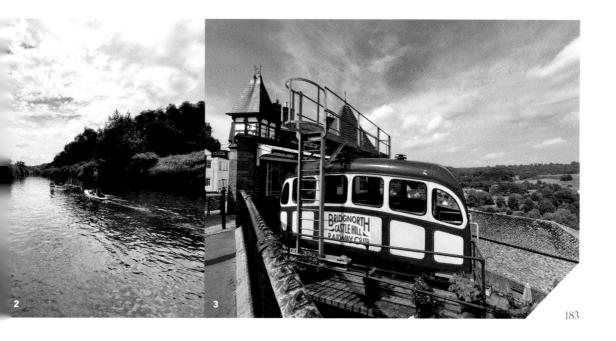

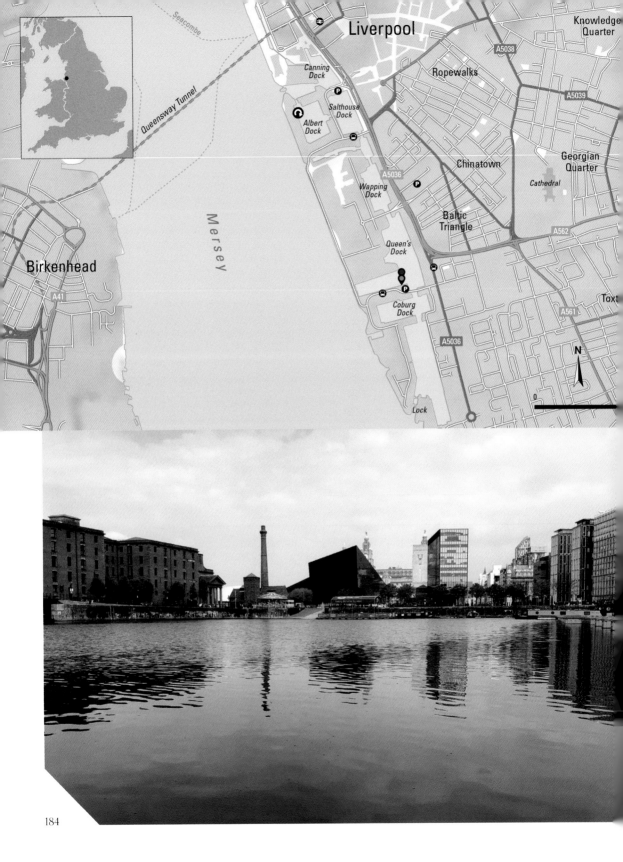

Royal Albert Dock, Liverpool

SUP IN THE CITY, THE LIVER BIRD WINGS, TATE LIVERPOOL AND THE WARMTH OF PEOPLE

It was the warmth of the light in Liverpool's Royal Albert Dock that first caught my eye. Researching my 2019 coast-to-coast adventure from Liverpool to Goole on Instagram, I was struck by the beauty of the deep-red brickwork and huge cast-iron columns reflected on the water. Sunset paddles following glitter trails framed not by ocean views but the Royal Liver Building and waterfront Museum of Liverpool.

I had never paddled in a city before. Would I find the tranquility I experience on the sea, I wondered? How self-conscious would I feel paddleboarding so close to people enjoying the bars on the boardwalk or visitors to Tate Liverpool? There was only one way to find out. It had been three years since my first SUP lesson and I was keen to improve my technical skills, so I booked a morning's one-on-one coaching with Jayne Rigby of Liverpool SUP Co, who runs her business from the Liverpool Watersports Centre in Queen's Dock. The centre is part of Local Solutions, a charity working with disadvantaged groups around the Liverpool city region and North Wales that are committed to making water sports accessible to everyone. It offers its own open-water swimming, kayaking, sailing and SUP classes.

Born and raised in Liverpool, Jayne fell in love with SUP in Jersey in 2015 and wanted to bring it home to the city she loves. She has a passion for the environment, and with her trusty Staffie Oscar she works with paddleboard brand Starboard SUP to bring communities and businesses from the city and surrounding coastline together for beach cleans and shoreline workshops on marine conservation.

We spent the morning on the Royal Albert Dock, building my confidence and technical skills, then had coffee and cake at 92 Degrees cafe while talking about our dreams. Jayne was contemplating leaving her post at a conservation charity to devote herself full time to her SUP business, and I was about to paddle 260 kilometres litter picking. Cliched as it may sound, perhaps the photos we took at Paul Curtis's famous Liver Bird Wings artwork on Jamaica Street in the Baltic Triangle helped us both take that next leap of faith.

Keen to share such an interesting place to SUP with you, I return one Wednesday morning to Liverpool to paddle with Jayne and her clients. Walking from the railway station to Queen's Dock, I notice a seagull trying to crack something with its beak on the cobbled paving. 'Oh dear, plastic litter,' I think, ready to spring into beach-cleaning mode. Thankfully, I am wrong: it is a mussel shell, many of which I later spy growing on the stone walls of the dock. Filter feeders, they eat by collecting tiny organisms from the water, cleaning and filtering at the same time. I also spot moon jellyfish and tiny fish in the dark but clear water. Looking closely from my board, I can see the historic tidal markings carved into the stone wall by the bridges.

Liverpool was granted World Heritage status from UNESCO in 2004, and was one of just 32 World Heritage Sites in the UK. Stretching from Albert Dock to Stanley Dock, it encompassed the historic commercial districts and Ropewalks area. Albert Dock features more Grade-I-listed buildings than anywhere else in the country.

It is just over a kilometre and a half to Salthouse Quay from the Liverpool Watersports Centre where we enter the Royal Albert Dock,

Opposite A stunning SUP in the city

which was built in 1846 and named after Albert, the consort of Queen Victoria. The Maritime Museum and International Slavery Museum are housed along the northern side of the dock. Opened in 2007, on the two hundredth anniversary of the abolition of the British slave trade, the International Slavery Museum is the only museum in the world dedicated to the history of the transatlantic slave trade, its legacy and the role played by the port of Liverpool and merchants of the day. In the far corner to our right is Tate Liverpool, which, along with Tate Modern, Tate Britain and Tate St Ives, houses the national collection of British art from 1500 to the present day, as well as international modern and contemporary art.

The architecture of the buildings is stunning.

As my friend Adya Misra, who I paddled with in Nottingham (p95) reminded me, it is hard to imagine while looking at this vibrancy today that in the early 1980s the dock was abandoned and full of silt before its major regeneration. The wonder I felt the first time paddling in such a historic place soon returns.

One of our group, Cat, whose personal confidence has grown immeasurably since she started SUP, is practising step back turns and falls into the water. Determined and focused, she is soon back on the board trying again. My concerns about being overlooked are dispelled: we are in a little world of our own.

'I don't quite know how I can portray the magic,' I say, soaking up the atmosphere and watching a cormorant fly in front of the iconic

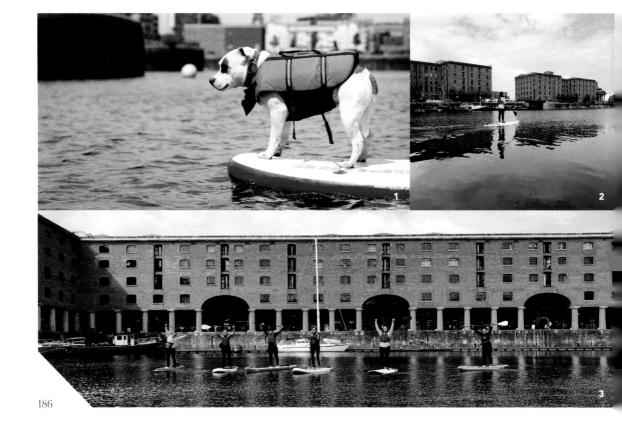

4 Going into Albert Dock

Royal Liver Building. Jayne smiles knowingly. I had wondered if paddleboarding in the dock would bring the calm I find on the sea and canals. As my shoulders drop and the tensions of the day float away, I realise I have answered my own question. Like Regent's Canal (p107) and Bristol Harbourside (p173), this is blue health in the city.

We paddle back to the Liverpool Watersports Centre, chatting side by side as Jayne offers encouragement and tips on technique. When I started SUP in 2016 there were fewer opportunities to build your skills after an initial beginner's lesson. Nowadays there are so many schools and freelance instructors that offer improver and progression classes, and I would highly recommend them.

I message Cat later to thank her for her time and inspiration, explaining how I'm trying to find the right words to describe paddleboarding in the Royal Albert Dock. 'I always think Liverpool stays in your heart,' she replies, 'you'll think of the words. They're inside you already.'

I realise immediately that she's right: paddleboarding in Liverpool is a unique city adventure. Whether you come simply to paddle in the docks alone or use it as a base to travel to the Lake District or North Wales, it is somewhere very special. It was the warmth of the light that drew me to the Royal Albert Dock. It is the beauty of the city and the warmth of the people that continue to bring me back. I hope you'll experience it too.

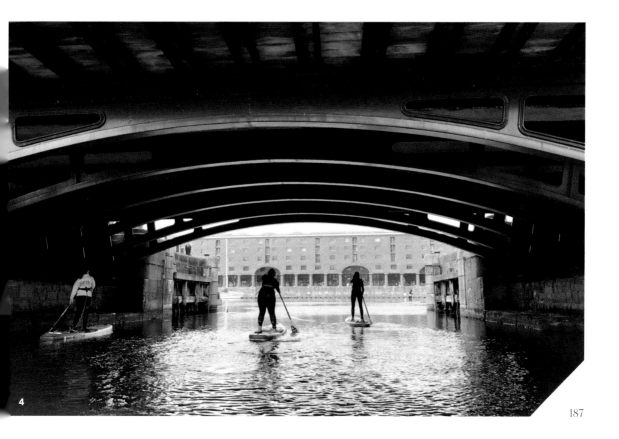

Technical Information

DISTANCE **3.2km round trip.**

LAUNCH LOCATION
ENTRY AND EXIT POINT **SJ 346889/53.393, -2.985**
TURN AROUND POINT **SJ 340898/53.401, -2.993**

Difficulty

This is a short paddle to the Royal Albert Dock and back and a good place to practise your technical skills. Be aware of kayakers, canoeists, boats and rowers that also use the docks.

Getting there

Liverpool is very accessible by rail, car or bus. The main railway station is Liverpool Lime Street (with connections to major cities including London and Manchester), a 2.5km walk to Liverpool Watersports Centre. There are two main bus stations: Liverpool One and Queen Square, with Stagecoach and National Express services arriving at Liverpool One, just over 1km away from the launch point. Buses from Liverpool Lime Street and throughout Liverpool can be caught within 300m of the launch point.

There is a car park by the Liverpool Watersports Centre (SJ 345888/53.392, -2.985) and plenty of pay-and-display car parks nearby.

Route information

To explore Albert Dock and launch from the Liverpool Watersports Centre independently (if you are experienced and have your own board) you need to buy a self-launch pass. Each person in a group must buy a pass, which is valid for four hours and can only be used once each day. You can hire boards, leashes and buoyancy aids, which must be worn. A monthly pass is also available.

Eating and drinking

» 92 Degrees serves coffee and cake.
» Carmine's Italian Cafe and Deli comes recommended from Jayne.

Instruction, guided tours and equipment hire

» Liverpool SUP Co offers lessons, tours and social SUP clubs.
» Liverpool Watersports Centre offers board hire and lessons.

Further information

» Paul Curtis Artwork: *www.paulcurtisartwork.com*
» Canal & River Trust have an audio walking tour from Royal Albert Dock to Stanley Dock: *www.canalrivertrust.org.uk/news-and-views/features/audio-tours/liverpool-link*

Opposite Paddling in Wapping Dock

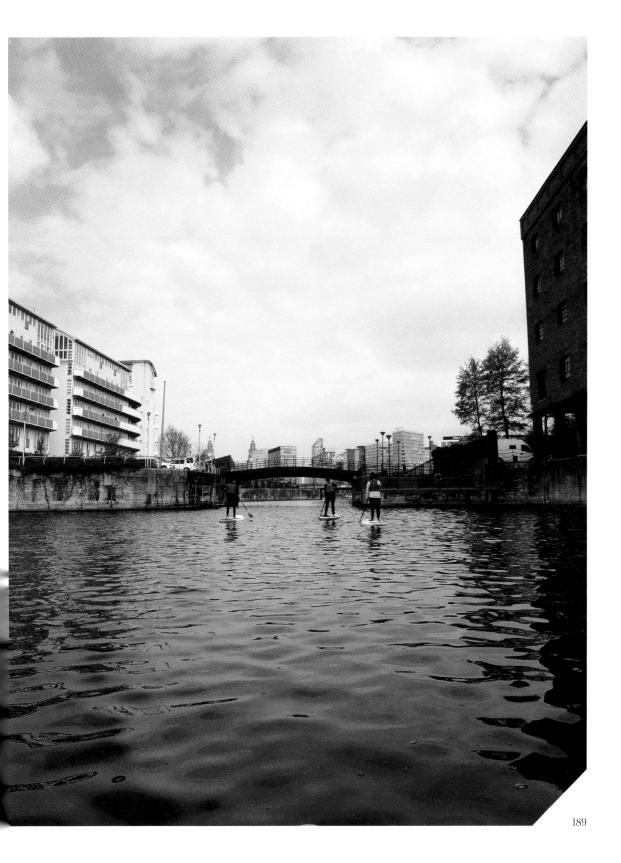

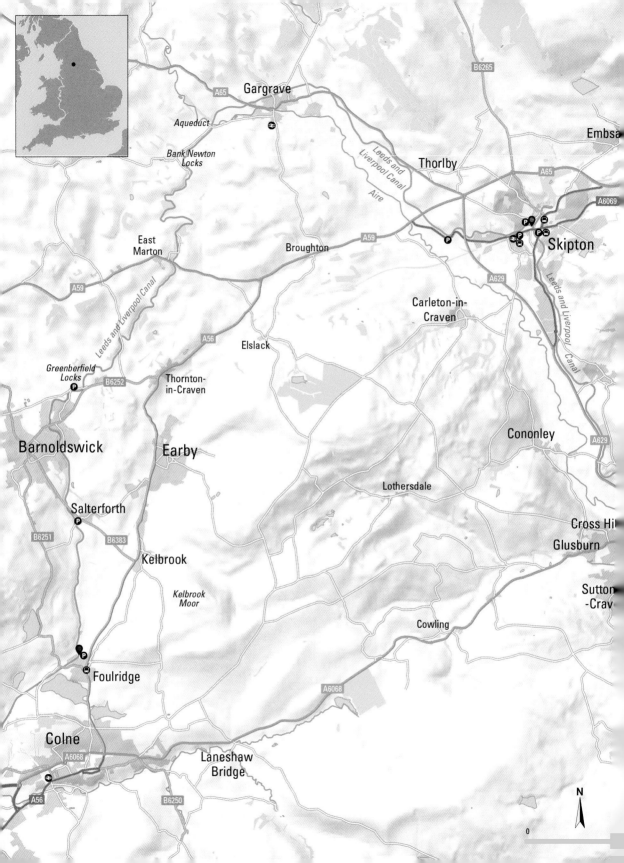

Skipton to Foulridge Tunnel, Leeds and Liverpool Canal

A GORGEOUS SUMMER'S DAY IN YORKSHIRE, FAIRY LIGHTS ON THE NARROWBOATS, A COW CALLED BUTTERCUP AND A FLOATING MUSEUM

The Leeds and Liverpool Canal will always hold a special place in my heart. In the summer of 2019, I paddleboarded the 260-kilometre coast-to-coast trail from Liverpool in the west to Goole in the east. The trail is made up of the Leeds and Liverpool Canal and the Aire and Calder Navigation. At just over 204 kilometres, the Leeds and Liverpool Canal is the longest canal in Britain built in a single waterway and was completed in 1816, 46 years after work began.

The adventure was a spark of a dream I had nurtured for three years as I built up my paddleboarding confidence. When I originally shared my idea in 2016, shortly after my first SUP lesson in the Lake District, the response was less than positive: I was told it would be logistically complex, possibly quite boring and too difficult for a woman of my age. I was 51 at the time.

The reality of the journey was very different: it became one of the most uplifting and joyful 11 days of my life as I paddled along this blue and green ribbon of the north. With 91 locks and 225 bridges – with some swing bridges so low I had to lie flat on my board, Grace, and swoosh under – the Leeds and Liverpool Canal passes through rural villages, urban housing estates, cities and fields of sheep. To SUP alongside moorhens and geese, listen to the curlews overhead and watch dragonflies gently land on my paddle whenever I felt weary was the greatest privilege. A summer's evening litter picking the flight of 21 locks in Wigan was magical. Memories of being caught in a

thunderstorm in Blackburn and chatting to a stranger as we took refuge under a bridge still make me smile. I came to understand how much the canal means to everyone who visits to fish, cycle, walk, run or cruise along in a narrowboat. It is a place to celebrate, contemplate, commiserate and seek sanctuary from daily life.

On 2 August 2019, I paddled 38 kilometres from Reedley Marina just outside Burnley to Skipton, arriving in my hometown at 10.30 p.m. as I paddled past fairy lights on the narrowboats, a towpath illuminating my way. It will remain one of the most treasured days of my life. From Skipton the canal then makes its way to Bingley Five Rise Locks, the steepest staircase of locks in the UK, and the UNESCO World Heritage Site of Saltaire.

The 26-kilometre route I'm sharing from Skipton to Foulridge was part of this special day (albeit in the opposite direction) and takes you through some of the most glorious countryside on the edge of the Yorkshire Dales and Lancashire. On a summer's afternoon it will feel like a little piece of heaven, with oystercatchers swooping above and butterflies dancing along the edge of the towpath. In autumn the leaves will be a golden backdrop to your journey.

Skipton, with its castle and bustling high street, was voted the second-happiest place to live in 2020 and will give you a warm welcome. On market days, you can stock up on fresh, local food before you set off from the pretty Skipton Canal Basin to Foulridge. If you fancy it, there's even a floating ice cream boat. You will paddle to Gargrave and then Bank Newton Locks, following the bends and curves of the canal with

1 Admiring reflections at near Gargrave   **2** One of the many stone bridges on the Leeds and Liverpool Canal

far-reaching views across the fields. Around 14 kilometres from Skipton you'll reach the double-arched bridge at East Marton. Next up is the highest point of the canal at Greenberfield Locks, where the historical *Kennet*, a floating interactive museum run by the Leeds and Liverpool Canal Society, has a mooring. Then onwards to Foulridge Tunnel. At just under a kilometre and a half long, it is an opportunity some of you might seize and others will, understandably, not. Local legend tells that in September 1912 a cow called Buttercup fell into the canal, swam right through the tunnel and was revived with brandy.

My experience 170 years later is less dramatic. The traffic-light system, in place so you don't meet oncoming boats, changes to green three minutes after I arrive at the entrance. While the idea of paddling a

kilometre and a half in the dark had played on my mind in the preceding months, I now don't have time to be scared. With my hooter, whistle and torches, I simply set forth and paddle as fast I could. The tunnel is so straight that you can see a tiny pinpoint at the other end as you enter, and there are three shafts of light that break up the darkness. Unlike Buttercup, 22 minutes later it is a nice cup of Yorkshire tea and flapjack that await me at the other end as I celebrate a tiny but momentous SUP achievement.

Whether you choose to add Foulridge Tunnel to your journey or step off the canal at The Wharf at Foulridge and head back to Skipton, this is truly a gorgeous route. I hope it brings you cherished moments and memories as it did for me. One definitely not to be missed.

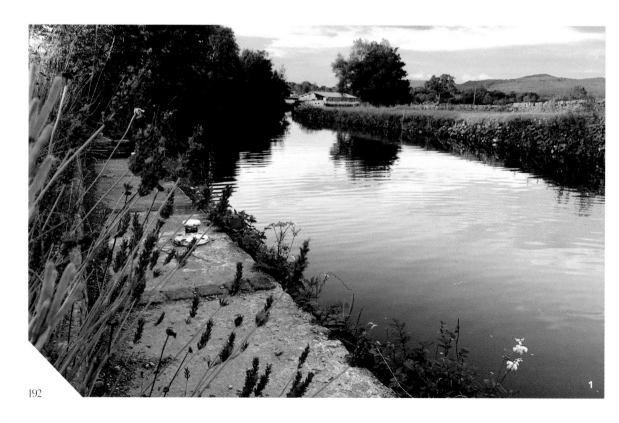

1

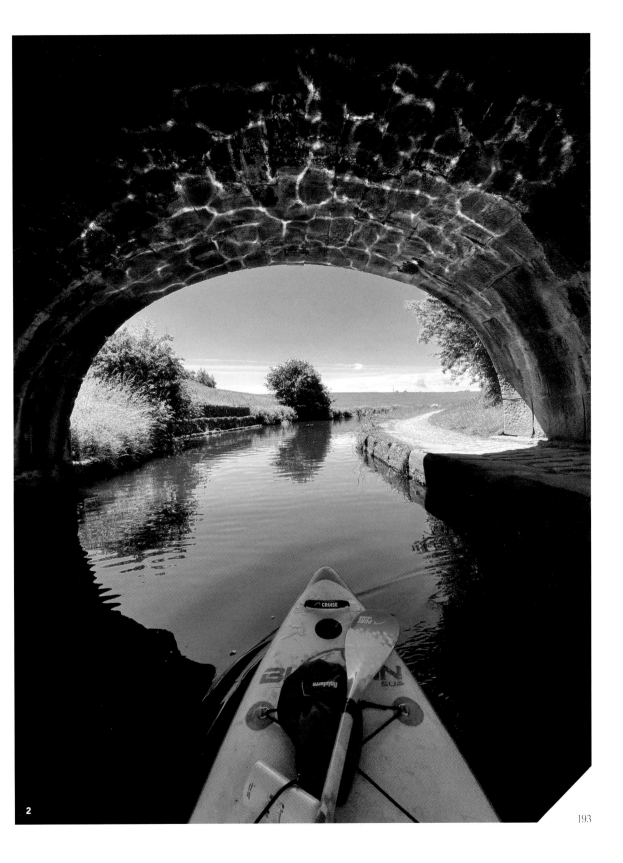

Technical information

DISTANCE **26km one way.**

LAUNCH LOCATION
ENTRY POINT **SD 988517/53.961, -2.020**
EXIT POINT **SD 889425/53.879, -2.171**

Difficulty
Paddleboarding on a canal has advantages for a beginner as you do not have to think about tides and river flow. It is often, but not always, more sheltered, and is a good place to build up skills. Things to consider are that portaging around locks means that you need to get off and back on to the canal. There are swing bridges which can be very low, which might require you to lie on your stomach to travel under, or you can portage around the bridge. It is also worth remembering that under a taller bridge, such as the lovely stone bridge at Gargrave, the wind is funnelled, so be aware of this or drop to your knees for stability. Also ensure you look out for narrowboats. If you do fall off, you are close to the towpath and the canal is often only waist-deep.

Getting there
Skipton is widely connected by rail, bus and car. The railway station, with connections to Leeds and Bradford, is 650m away from the launch point. The bus station, with services to Ilkley, Settle and other local towns, is 500m away.

Parking is available at the railway station (SD 983514/53.959, -2.026), Coach Street (SD 987517/53.962, -2.020), Cavendish Street (SD 988515/53.959, -2.020) and Bridge Street (SD 987517/53.961, -2.021) car parks within a few hundred metres of the canal basin. Bridge Street car park has public toilets.

Foulridge is just off the A56, as 17km drive from Skipton. Turn right at the Causeway and there are signs to Foulridge Wharf. There is ample free parking next to The Wharf at Foulridge restaurant (SD 889426/53.880, -2.171).

If you'd prefer to paddle one way and take the bus back to Skipton, the Pendle Wizz bus from Burnley stops at Foulridge, 500m from the exit point.

Parking is available at Skipton, as well as a few spaces along the canal if you would like to break up the route: Niffany Bridge (SD 969514/53.958, -2.048), Greenberfield Locks (SD 888482/53.930, -2.173) and Salterforth (SD 888454/53.904, -2.172).

Staying in Skipton
As this is a longer route than most, I am including places to stay if you would like to break up the journey. There are lots of places to stay in Skipton and along the route right on the canal:

» Herriots Hotel and the Hotel Rendezvous in Skipton.
» Niffany Farm Caravan and Camping is 1.5km outside Skipton.
» Anchor Inn Cookhouse & Pub and Premier Inn at Gargrave are 8km from Skipton.
» Newton Grange holiday cottages are 11km along the canal from Skipton. The beautiful farm backs right on to the canal, and staying here would allow you to paddle in either direction and explore the canal across a few days. You can even see the canal bridge from your bedroom window.

Route information
A Waterways Licence is required for this route.

Bridge numbers start at number one in Liverpool, rising towards Leeds. Lock numbers start at number one in Leeds, rising towards Liverpool.

The Foulridge Tunnel on the Leeds and Liverpool Canal is open all year round. For safety, it operates a traffic-light system. Heading towards Leeds, entering from the westerly portal, the light will be green for 10 minutes on the half an hour. Heading towards Liverpool,

1 Greenberfield Locks   **2** The double-arched bridge at East Marton

entering from the easterly portal, the light will be green for 10 minutes on the hour.

Start paddleboarding through the tunnel when the green light is shown. I'm not a particularly fast paddleboarder, so 30 minutes should be plenty. I recommend going on your knees and taking torches and a whistle, which will let people know that you are coming. If on the day there is a fault with the light, let the Canal & River Trust North West customer support team know by calling 03030 404040.

Eating and drinking

» Steep&Filter refill shop in Skipton is an independent coffee house, refill shop and greengrocers. It sells delicious bread, vegetables and fruit – and the best Tony's Chocolonely chocolate – for a picnic on your board.
» Elsworth Kitchen in Skipton offers a platter box or cake takeaway, which you can order ahead for a sumptuous SUP treat.
» The seasonal Lock Stop cafe at Greenberfield Locks serves hot butties and homemade cakes as well as teas and coffees from a wooden cabin, a stone's throw from the canal.
» The Anchor Inn at Salterforth is a pub and restaurant right by bridge 151. It offers

picnic boxes and takeaway drinks as well as pub classics.
» The Wharf at Foulridge serves hot drinks, cakes, tapas and salads right on the canal edge in a beautiful old wharf building. It also has live music evenings.

Instruction, guided tours and equipment hire

» This is a route for those who have their own boards as there are currently no opportunities for hiring or lessons on this stretch.
» For lessons in North Yorkshire, try Learn to Paddle, SUP Active Yorkshire or Lost Earth Adventures.

Further information

» Find out more about the history of the canal with the Leeds and Liverpool Canal Society and their floating museum boat, *Kennet*:
www.leedsandliverpoolcanalsociety.co.uk
» The Collins/Nicholson Waterways guidebooks are very helpful if you are considering paddleboarding on canals. For this area, look for *North West & the Pennines: Waterways Guide 5* (Nicholson, 2015).

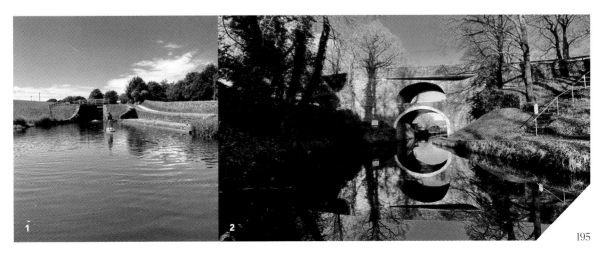

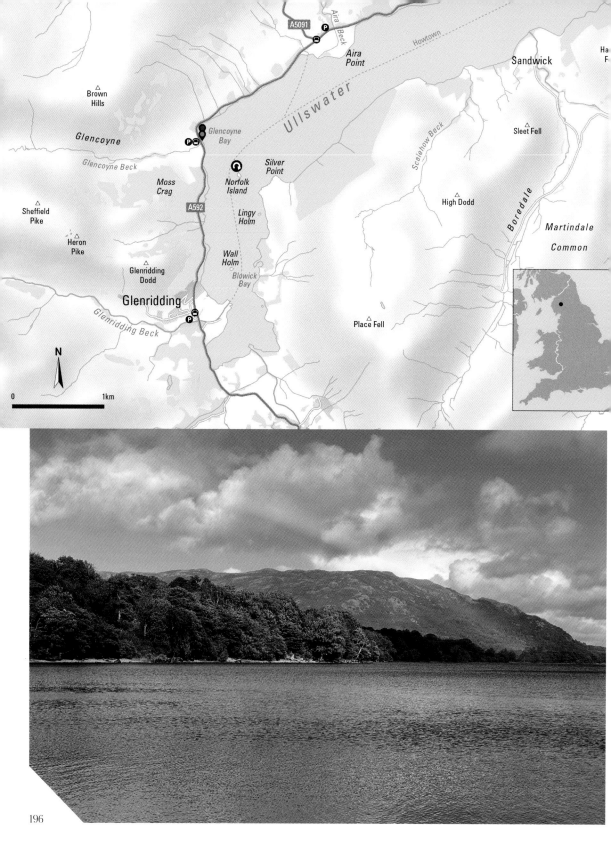

Ullswater

**A RAINBOW OVER THE LAKE, ULLSWATER
STEAMERS, A WANDERLUST WOMAN AND
DREAMING OF DAFFODILS**

'Oh, wow, look at the rainbow over the lake.'

It's an afternoon on the cusp between late
summer and early autumn and I'm pumping
up my board on the shores of Ullswater, the
second-largest body of water in the Lake
District National Park in the north-west of
England. Adventurer Amira Patel, also known
as the Wanderlust Woman, and I have just
arrived at Glencoyne Bay to paddle together.
We pause, taking in the beauty ahead of us.
A serendipitous moment to cherish.

Writing this book has felt like writing a love
letter to the beautiful places on our doorstep,
our sport and the paddleboarding community
that makes it so special. When my head was
bursting with facts and maps, I added a note
in my journal: 'let the research breathe. Leave
space for serendipity.' This was a lesson I
learned when crossing coast to coast in 2019.
Chance meetings, the kindness of strangers and
magical meteorological moments along the
canal enriched that experience in ways I could
neither have expected nor engineered.

I'm grateful that serendipity has also played
a part in the journey of this book. There have
been times of wonder: dolphins swimming past,
watching an otter feed on the rocks and
a curious seal choosing to swim under my
board. I've shared breathtaking sunrises and
sunsets, the glassiest of waters along the coast
and, with just the right amount of wind behind
our backs, a few minutes whooshing along
the water, laughing. The generosity of new
friends sharing their knowledge and time has
moved me to tears. There have of course been
cancelled days, grey days and rainy days, as you

have read. There have been rainbows too.

Now, unexpectedly, due to schedules falling
through and plans postponed because of
forecasted winds, I am in the Lake District once
again to conclude my research. After travelling
across England, Scotland and Wales, I am
preparing to launch less than 32 kilometres from
where I took my first SUP lesson a few years
before. I have come full circle back to where my
love for paddleboarding began. Serendipity, my
old friend.

At just under 12 kilometres long, just over
a kilometre across and 62 metres at its deepest,
Ullswater is described both as a ribbon across
the countryside and a stretched 'Z' shape. It has
three distinct sections, or reaches, formed by
three different glaciers.

The village of Pooley Bridge, originally
named 'Pooley' or 'Pool How' meaning the hill
beside the pool, stands at the northern tip of
Ullswater, overlooked by Dunmallet. Glenridding
sits at the south, backed by Helvellyn, the
third-highest mountain within the Lake District
and England. The Ullswater Valley is also an
important place for farming the distinctive
Herdwick sheep. The two villages are connected
on the water by the Ullswater Steamers,
in operation since 1859. They also stop at
Howtown Pier on the eastern shore and Aira
Force Waterfall on the north-western. For a small
fee, the company will carry a limited number
of deflated paddleboards, which is something
to consider if you'd like to paddle one way
and enjoy a ride on MY *Lady of the Lake* or MV
Western Belle on your return. The magnificent
Aira Force, home not only to a 20-metre
waterfall drop but also to a population of native
red squirrels, is two and a half kilometres from
where Amira and I are watching the rainbow.

Opposite The view from Glencoyne Bay

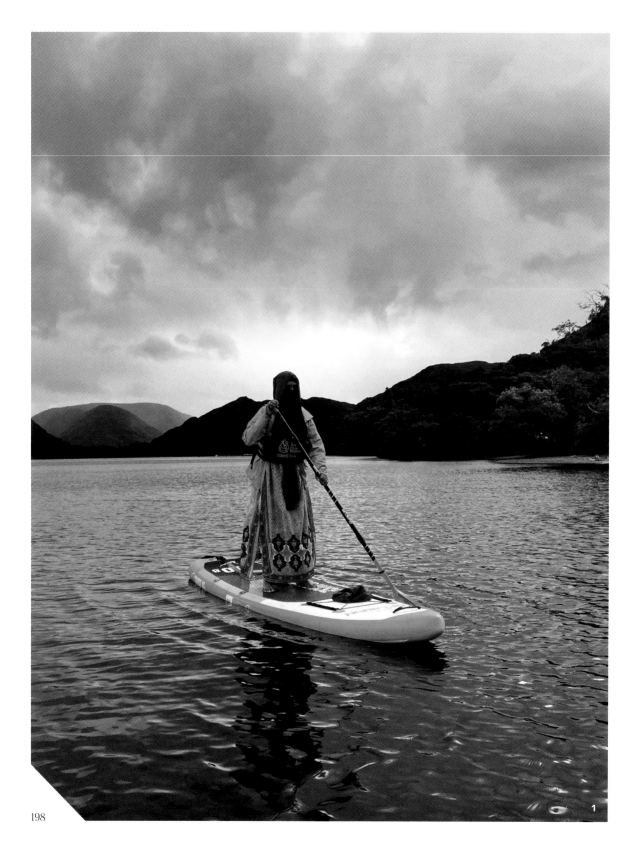

1

1 Amira making her way into Glencoyne Bay   **2** Looking towards Silver Crag

I first met Amira, founder of The Wanderlust Women, a hiking and adventure group for Muslim women, in spring at Sheffield Adventure Film Festival. Her film about her love of the outdoors, *The Wanderlust Women*, which also features her mum Aysha Yilmaz, was directed by my friend Frit Tam and touched me deeply. We swapped numbers and made tentative plans to paddleboard together in the Lakes, where she now lives.

With her mum's encouragement, Amira has always loved adventure, and as a young girl enjoyed hiking and cycling. Years later, after her divorce, she found the mountains helped her heal. It was there she rediscovered her courage and self-belief, learning to kayak, climb and SUP. As she works towards her Mountain Leader qualification, her vision is to encourage other Muslim women to feel confident and represented in nature. She organises hikes, well-being retreats and outdoor training,

alongside her photography, speaking and consultancy work.

Our launch point is a small beach just a few careful steps from the National Trust Glencoyne car park across a busy road. Within minutes, we meet hikers and wild swimmers enjoying the lake and admiring the views and families of swans.

Over two centuries before, it was at Glencoyne Bay that Dorothy Wordsworth and her brother, the poet William Wordsworth, saw the spring daffodils by the lake on 15 April 1802, while walking back to Grasmere from Pooley Bridge. In her journal, Dorothy wrote:

'I never saw daffodils so beautiful they grew among the mossy stones about and about them, some rested their heads upon these stones as on a pillow for weariness and the rest tossed and reeled and danced and seemed as if they verily laughed with the wind that blew upon them over the lake, they looked so gay

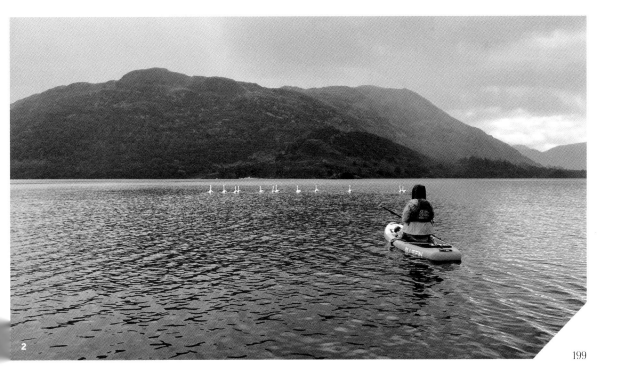

ever dancing ever changing. This wind blew directly over the lake to them. There was here and there a little knot and a few stragglers a few yards higher up but they were so few as not to disturb the simplicity and unity and life of that one busy highway. We rested again and again. The Bays were stormy, and we heard the waves at different distances and in the middle of the water like the sea.'

Two years later, William wrote his poem *I Wandered Lonely as a Cloud* recalling this walk together. It was published in 1807 and is now one of England's most famous and best-loved poems.

The lake is not stormy today but we are mindful of the clouds and the wind, especially as we watch a paddler working hard ahead of us. We edge our way towards Norfolk Island, which lies between Glencoyne and Silver Point, and then turn back to the shelter of the bay. We chat about friendship and belonging and the power of nature to heal, uplift and bring people together. Paddling side by side, close to the shore and in a world of our own, we enjoy 45 minutes of gentle paddleboarding. Today is less about distance covered and more about joy experienced and ideas exchanged. The outdoors is Amira's office now, and what an office she has welcomed me to: bright-blue skies one minute, rain the next; mountains, lush trees, islands and the clear waters of the lake.

With Amira's delicious picnic by my side, I leave Ullswater with a full heart and journal bursting with ideas for the future. It is a truly beautiful place to SUP, and while today may mark the beginning of the end of my research for this book, it will not be my last paddleboarding trip here. It is time for the next chapter. I'm already planning an adventure from Glenridding to Pooley Bridge with friends in spring, when the daffodils Dorothy and William Wordsworth so beautifully described are blooming once again. Perhaps we will see you there? I hope so.

Technical Information

DISTANCE **1.6km round trip.**
LAUNCH LOCATION ENTRY AND EXIT POINT **NY 387188/54.561, -2.949** TURN AROUND POINT **NY 391185/54.558, -2.943**

Difficulty

Paddling further out and along the length of Ullswater would require experience and an understanding of the wind; it can whip up quickly and create waves on the water. The prevailing wind is from the southwest and would usually (but not always) blow up the lake from Glenridding. Hug the shoreline for shelter. Be aware that the water in Ullswater can be very cold and dress accordingly.

Glencoyne Bay is quite sheltered for a beginner in the right conditions.

Getting there

Ullswater is considered one of the most easily accessible lakes. Penrith is approximately 10km from the northern tip of Ullswater. The nearest railway station is Penrith, 19km from the launch point. A bus runs from Penrith to Pooley Bridge, Aira Force and Glenridding and also stops just by the launch point. On holidays and weekends, a bus runs from Keswick to Aira Force and Glenridding, should you wish to travel to Derwent Water.

The launch point is 17km from junction 40 on the M6. Glencoyne Bay car park is a pay and display (NY 387189/54.561, -2.950). Parking is free for National Trust members. There are free car parking spaces along the A592 which borders the lake, although these can fill up quickly.

Route information

The Glenridding Hotel and the Quiet Site holiday park are the closest webcams.

1 Just before we set off

Eating and drinking

I bought a picnic from the famous Tebay Services Farmshop and Kitchen on the M6 and Amira gave me another!

» Verey Books in Pooley Bridge sells wonderful books, as well as hot drinks and cakes.
» The National Trust Aira Force Tea Room sells sandwiches, hot drinks and cakes.
» Rheged Cafe is just under 2km from junction 40 of the M6 and 17km from Glencoyne car park.

Instruction, guided tours equipment hire

» Ullswater Paddleboarding offers lessons, paddleboard hire and guided tours of Ullswater, including a short one from Glencoyne Bay and a longer, full-length tour of the lake.
» Lake District Paddle Boarding offers lessons and guided tours of Ullswater.
» Another Place, The Lake offers SUP tuition for guests with Ullswater Paddleboarding.

Further information

» The Wanderlust Women: *www.instagram.com/the.wanderlust.women/?hl=en*
» Ullswater Steamers: *www.ullswater-steamers.co.uk*
» Tebay Services Farmshop and Kitchen at junction 38 on the M6 offers a farm shop, cafe, hotel, showers and fuel: *www.tebayservices.com*
» Eden Rivers Trust have an excellent guide on paddling the whole of Ullswater: *www.edenriverstrust.org.uk*
» The Lake District is very popular so check the Lake District car parking forecast during holidays: *www.lakedistrict.gov.uk*
» Check the Lake District Weatherline in addition to your usual weather planning: *www.lakedistrictweatherline.co.uk*
» Suzanna Cruickshank, *Swimming Wild in the Lake District: The most beautiful wild swimming spots in the larger Lakes* (Vertebrate Publishing, 2020).

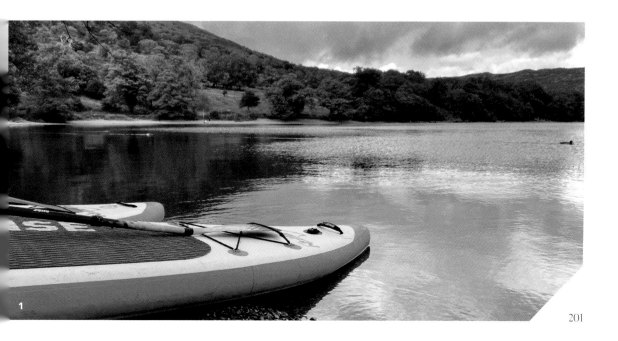

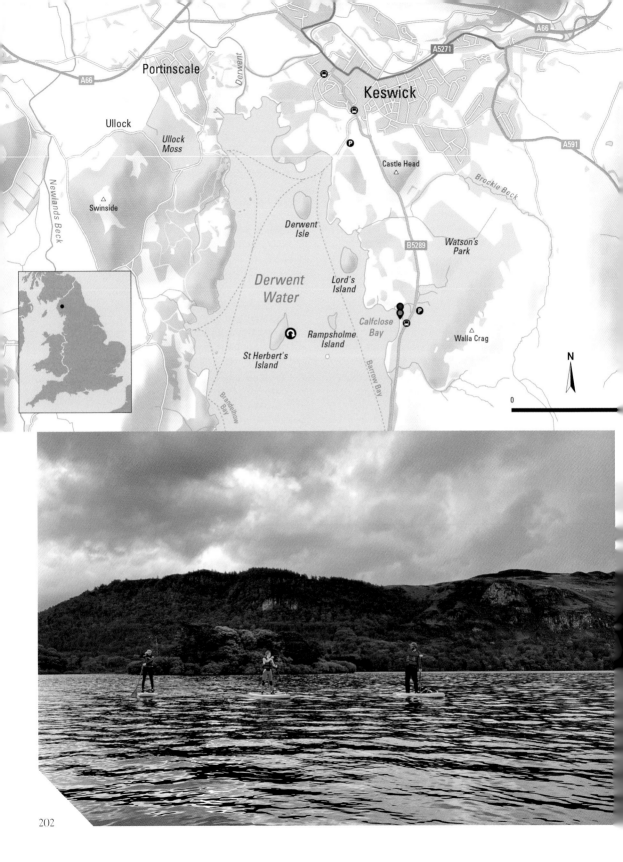

Derwent Water

SWALLOWS AND AMAZONS, BEATRIX POTTER, MAGNIFICENT MOUNTAINS AND THE HUNDRED YEAR STONE

Diary entry, 24 September 2016: 'Dreams do come true! 1st paddleboarding lesson in the Lakes. I loved it!'

One of the questions I ask all of my guests on *The Joy of SUP – The Paddleboarding Sunshine Podcast* is, 'Do you remember how you felt the first time you went on a paddleboard?' I love hearing their answers – they feature joy, uncertainty, excitement, courage, freedom, triumph and, yes, that moment when perhaps it didn't go quite as planned. There is a connection, a shared experience across the airwaves. I understand all those feelings as I recall the overcast afternoon in 2016 when I travelled to Derwent Water in the Lake District National Park in the north-west of England for my first paddleboarding lesson. Today that tiny but significant entry, written next to the note to review my home insurance and the date for parents' evening, always makes me smile.

After injuring my knee in January 2016, I had been in pain for some time and my usual enthusiasm for life had been knocked. As my knee healed, I set myself a challenge on 1 September to spend 30 minutes each day moving outside, to lift my spirits and strengthen my leg. Having researched the benefits of paddleboarding for our physical and mental well-being and, I'll admit, being attracted by the aspirational photos of blue waters and sunny locations online, a SUP lesson was a treat on the horizon. I arrived on the edge of Derwent Water to meet Bo from Lake District Paddle Boarding with such hope and a childlike enthusiasm to learn everything I could. After our safety and kit introduction,

we launched on to the water near the Derwent Water Marina on the north-west shore.

I will not pretend that I was super confident or skilful. Learning something new as an adult is always a little nerve-wracking. What I was certain of within minutes, however, was that paddleboarding was something very special. As I looked out across Derwent Water, standing momentarily with a sense of calm, I exhaled deeply with my head up, my shoulders back and my heart full. For the first time in months I felt like a warrior, not a worrier. I couldn't stop smiling for days. Two months later I travelled to Southport, and as hail began to fall on the Marine Lake I paddled on a few different boards with Alan from SUP North UK. My teeth were chattering and I could barely feel my fingers as I changed by the roadside, but it didn't matter. Just shy of my fifty-second birthday I became a paddleboarder.

Writing my list of beautiful places to share with you, the Lake District was an immediate choice not only because of this deep personal connection but also because for many paddleboarders it has become a favourite destination. With stunning scenery, wildlife and history it is not difficult to see why. The Lake District is the largest national park in England at 583,747 acres. It is made up of 13 valleys, and in July 2017 became a UNESCO World Heritage Site. Within the park there are 16 lakes, although Bassenthwaite Lake is in fact the only official lake, the rest being meres or waters. Windermere is the largest lake and is also the longest in England at just under 17 kilometres, and Wast Water is the deepest lake in England at 79 metres. It includes 42 kilometres of coastline and estuaries, and 12 per cent of the national park is covered by

Opposite On our way to St Herbert's Island

woodland. At 978 metres, Scafell Pike is the highest mountain.

It's a sunny, late-spring day as I meet John Wilson, who founded Lake District Paddle Boarding in 2014 after his own adventure paddling from the Lake District to the Irish Sea with Simon Palmer of SUP Adventures, mentioned in my Runswick Bay chapter (p89). We didn't meet back in 2016 but I am keen to thank him and Bo for quite simply changing my life.

An hour later, after driving to Great Wood car park, one of John's team, Mick Stockdale, and I launch from Calfclose Bay into a slight breeze, heading out towards Rampsholme Island and on towards St Herbert's Island. Derwent Water is the third-largest lake in the Lake District and is four and a half kilometres long, just under two kilometres at its widest and 22 metres at its deepest, and is fed by the River Derwent in the south. A walk of a few hundred metres from the north-eastern shore lies Keswick, which contains lots of lovely cafes, the Derwent Pencil Museum, The Puzzling Place (a favourite when my boys were young) and Keswick Museum, which covers the landscape, social history of the area and the work of local artists. By the shore is the Theatre by the Lake, and nearby lie the jetties for the Keswick Launch Company, which offers cruises in beautiful wooden boats around the lake with eight hop-on, hop-off landings.

It is one of these boats that passes ahead of us as we make our way from the shore to the islands ahead. John had reminded me of them and I crouch to steady myself in the ensuing wake. Rampsholme Island is the smallest of the four main islands on Derwent Water, the other three being St Herbert's Island, Derwent Isle and Lord's Island, which are cared for by the

National Trust. Rampsholme Island's name is derived from the Old Norse word *hrafns holmr*, or wild garlic island.

The wind begins to pick up a little and a few minutes later we find ourselves paddling in quite a downpour. This is a timely reminder that while stunningly beautiful, it is always wise to be mindful of the wind and weather forecast when planning an adventure in the Lakes, and to prepare your clothing and kit accordingly. I'm grateful to be wearing a drysuit today.

We approach St Herbert's Island and Mick suggests we land and explore. The island is the largest of the four main islands on the lake, approximately four to five acres in size, and is named after Saint Herbert, who lived here as a hermit, growing vegetables and eating fish from the lake. If, like me, you grew up reading Beatrix Potter's books, you may know the island from the illustrations of her 1903 *The Tale of Squirrel Nutkin*. The National Trust even has a photo of her sketching on its shores. A passionate campaigner for conservation and friend of Canon Hardwicke Drummond Rawnsley, one of the three founding members of the charity, Potter bequeathed the National Trust 4,000 acres of land and countryside and 15 farms upon her death in 1943.

As we leave I comment that it all feels very *Swallow and Amazons*, with the lush, green trees and time to explore. 'You're right,' says Mick, 'the 2016 adaptation was filmed just here.'

The sun is shining once more, and as we paddle along Mick points out the 451-metre Cat Bells on the western shore, the 931-metre Skiddaw to the north of Keswick and Lord's Island, which was once the residence of the Earls of Derwent Water. To protect the wildlife such as the nesting geese that now call it home, the National Trust asks that no one lands

1 A break at Borrowdale   2 Heading towards St Herbert's Island   3 Aldis and Baiba
4 Taking in the views   5 The Hundred Year Stone

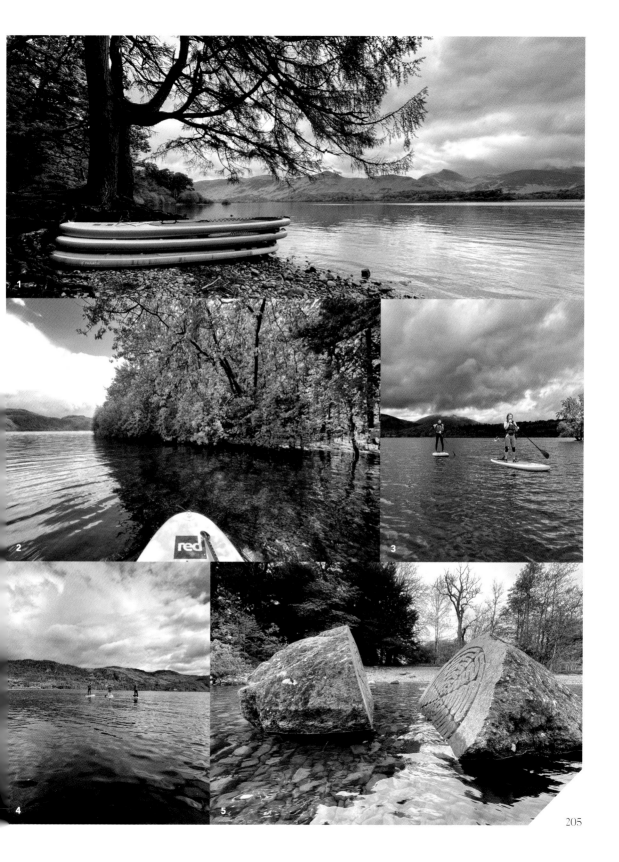

1 Looking out from St Herbert's Island
Overleaf Pure happiness near Newton Grange Farm, Skipton to Foulridge Tunnel © Guy Carpenter

here and that we respect a 'no-paddle' zone between the shoreline and island. The fourth island, Derwent Isle, is the only inhabited island and landing is not permitted. However, for five days a year the house and grounds are open to visitors via special canoe trips.

Returning to Calfclose Bay, our final stop is the Hundred Year Stone, a geometric sculpture carved from glacial boulder (andesite) from Borrowdale by Peter Randall-Page to commemorate the centenary of the National Trust. At different times of the year, the water levels reveal or cover the stone, and today we are able to paddle close and study the intricate beauty of the carving. A beautiful end to a lovely adventure.

Mountains, islands, forest bathing, history and art, there is so much beauty to explore on Derwent Water. The joy I felt when I first looked out on to the lake in 2016 has only grown with time. It will always have such a special place in my heart. I hope it will for you too.

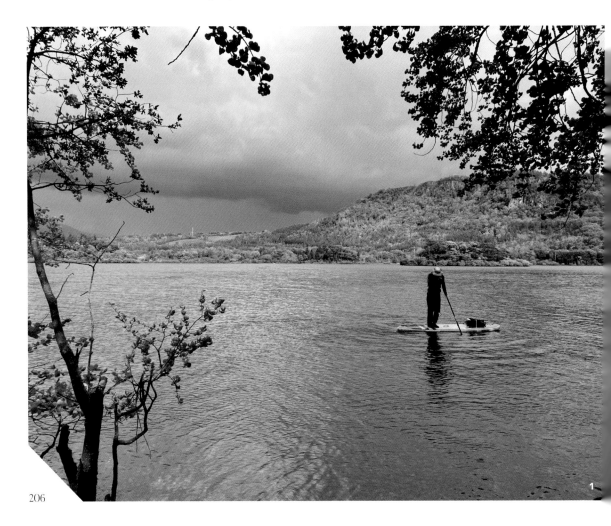

1

Tecnical information

DISTANCE **4km round trip.**

LAUNCH LOCATION
ENTRY AND EXIT POINT **NY 270214/54.582, -3.131**
TURN AROUND POINT **NY 260212/54.580, -3.146**

Difficulty

Paddling in the Lakes is always subject to the wind, so be aware of the conditions. Calfclose Bay is quite sheltered for a beginner in the right conditions. Be aware of the Keswick Launch Company and keep out of their way.

Getting there

The nearest railway station is Penrith, which is 29km from Keswick. Buses run from Penrith to Keswick every hour. If you are able to carry your board, you could take the bus from Seatoller to Keswick, which stops just by the launch point.

Keswick is 27km from junction 40 on the M6. Great Wood car park is a National Trust car park 3km outside of Keswick which is free to members (NY 272214/ 54.583, -3.128). You will need to cross and walk along a very busy road from the car park to the shore so do be careful. Alternatively the Theatre by the Lake has parking (NY 266229/54.596, -3.138).

Route information

Derwent Water Marina has a webcam.

Remember to Check, Clean and Dry your equipment and kit if paddleboarding on different Lakes in the Lake District to prevent the spread of invasive non-native species.

Eating and drinking

» There are lots of cafes in nearby Keswick.
» Theatre by the Lake serves brunch and lunch.
» Fellpack comes recommended by Suzanna Cruickshank in *Swimming Wild in the Lake District.*
» The Wild Strawberry has some great cakes.

Instruction, guided tours equipment hire

» Lake District Paddle Boarding offers lessons and guided tours of Derwent Water.
» Derwent Water Marina offers paddleboard hire and paddleboards for sale.

Further information

» Keswick Launch Company offer cruises and boat hire: *www.keswick-launch.co.uk*
» Tebay Services Farmshop and Kitchen at junction 38 on the M6 offers a farm shop, cafe, hotel, showers and fuel. It is great for picnics: *www.tebayservices.com*
» Check the Lake District Weatherline in addition to your usual weather planning: *www.lakedistrictweatherline.co.uk*
» Check the Lake District car parking forecast during holidays: *www.lakedistrict.gov.uk*
» Suzanna Cruickshank, *Swimming Wild in the Lake District: The most beautiful wild swimming spots in the larger Lakes* (Vertebrate Publishing, 2020).

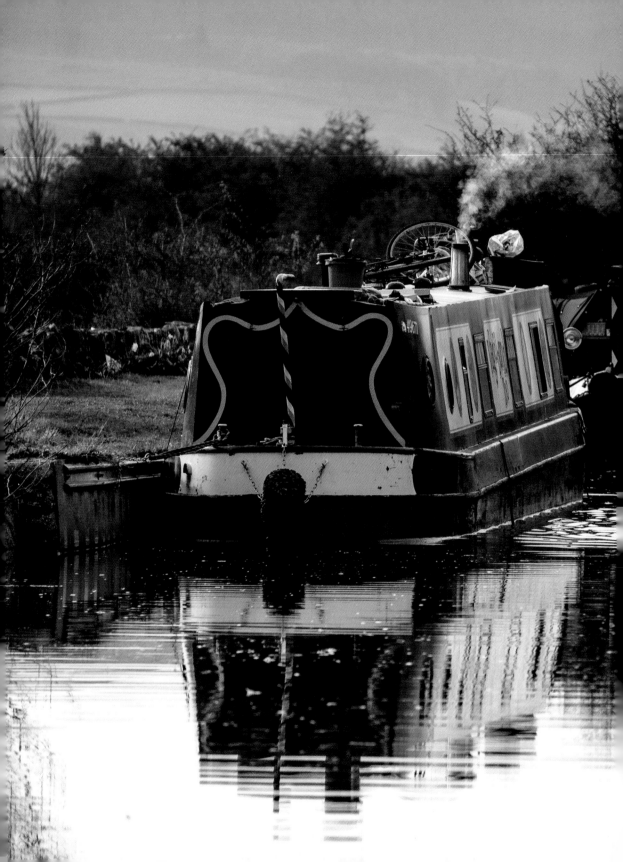

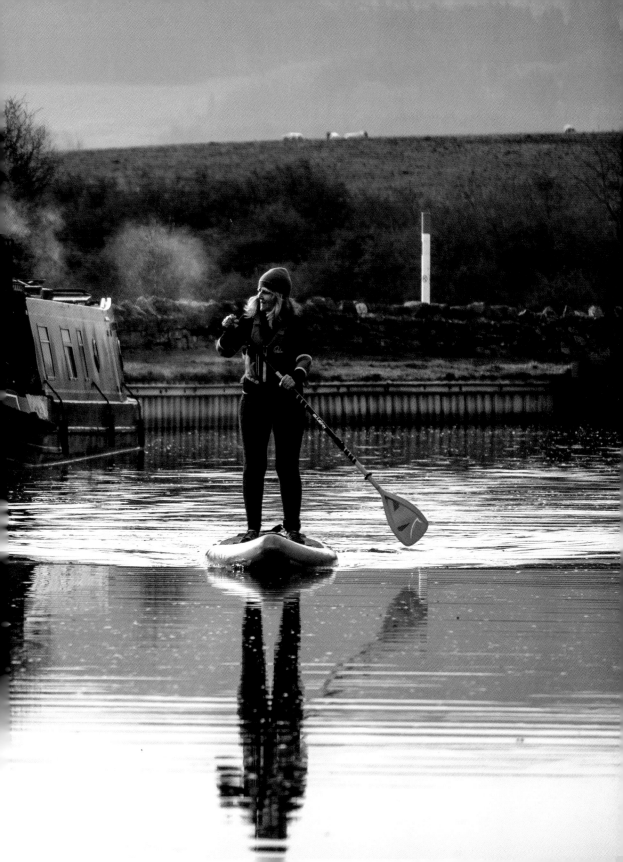

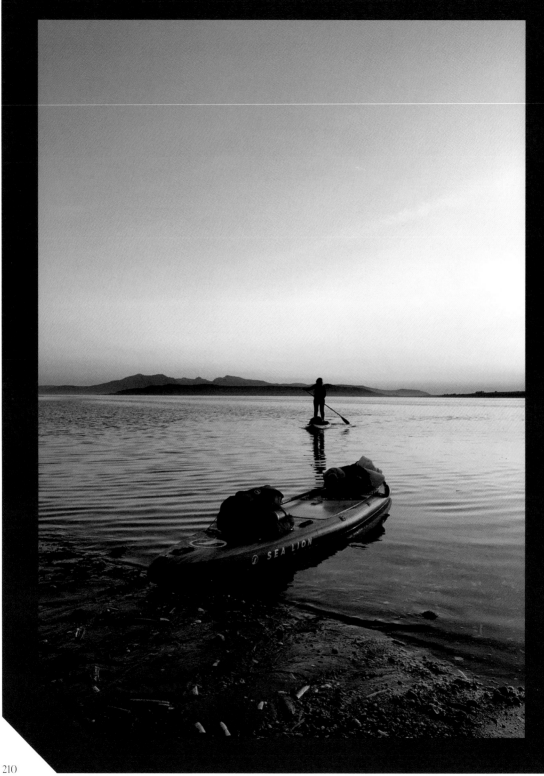

Further reading, listening and watching

Books

Admiralty Tidal Stream Atlas
United Kingdom Hydrographic Office

Canoe & Kayak Map of Britain
Peter Knowles
Rivers Publishing UK, 2014

Inland Waterways Map of Great Britain
Nicholson, 2020

North West & the Pennines: Waterways guide 5
Collins Maps
Nicholson, 2015

The Canal Guide: Britain's 50 best canals
Stuart Fisher
Adlard Coles, 2015

Great Glen Canoe Trail: A complete guide to Scotland's first formal canoe trail
Donald Macpherson
Pesda Press, 2020

How to Increase Your Stand Up Paddling Performance: Beginner to elite
Suzie Cooney
Suzie Trains Maui, 2015

Paddle the Thames: A guide for canoes, kayaks and SUPs
Mark Rainsley
Pesda Press, 2017

Paddling Britain: 50 best places to explore by SUP, kayak & canoe
Lizzie Carr
Bradt Travel Guide, 2018

Scottish SUP Guide: Where to stand up paddleboard in Scotland
Matt Gambles
Self-published, 2020

The SUP Book: How to stand up paddleboard
Matt Gambles
Self-published, 2020

Stand Up Paddle: A paddlers' guide
Steve West
Batini Books, 2012

Stand Up Paddleboarding: A beginner's guide
Simon Bassett
Fernhurst Books Ltd, 2019

Stand Up Paddling: Flatwater to surf and rivers
Rob Casey
Mountaineers Books, 2011

The Paddleboard Bible: The complete guide to stand up paddleboarding
Dave Price
Adlard Coles, 2021

Scottish Island Bagging: The Walkhighlands guide to the islands of Scotland
Helen and Paul Webster
Vertebrate Publishing, 2019

Swimming Wild in the Lake District: The most beautiful wild swimming spots in the Lake District
Suzanna Cruickshank
Vertebrate Publishing, 2020

The Beaches of Scotland: A selected guide to over 150 of the most beautiful beaches on the Scottish mainland and islands
Stacey McGowan Holloway
Vertebrate Publishing, 2022

The Beaches of Wales: The complete guide to every beach and cove around the Welsh coastline
Alistair Hare
Vertebrate Publishing, 2020

Water Ways: A thousand miles along Britain's canals
Jasper Winn
Profile Books Ltd, 2020

Ignore the Fear: One woman's paddleboarding adventure, 800 miles from Land's End to John O'Groats with a fear of the sea
Fiona Quinn
Lemon Publishing, 2019

Microadventures: Local discoveries for great escapes
Alastair Humphreys
William Collins, 2014

Move!: The new science of body over mind
Caroline Williams
Profile Books Ltd, 2021

Opposite A sunset SUP to Great Cumbrae, Portencross and Largs, the Cumbraes © @microadventuregirl

No. More. Plastic.: What you can do to make a difference
Martin Dorey
Ebury Press, 2018

The Book of Tides: A journey through the coastal waters of our island
William Thomson
Quercus Publishing, 2016

How To Read Water: Clues & patterns from puddles to the sea
Tristan Gooley
Sceptre, 2017

Water Gypsies: A history of life on Britain's rivers and canals
Julian Dutton
The History Press, 2021

Wild Waters: A wildlife and water lover's companion to the aquatic world
Susanne Masters
Vertebrate Publishing, 2022

Crossing the Bar – Tales of Wells Harbour
Robert Smith MBE
Self-published, 2018

We Bought an Island
Evelyn E Atkins
Polperro Heritage Press, 2010

Tales from Our Cornish Island: The story, sequel to We Bought an Island, of a dream that was made to come true
Evelyn E Atkins
Coronet Books, 1987

Websites and resources

British Canoeing: *www.britishcanoeing.org.uk*
British Stand Up Paddle Association (BSUPA): *www.bsupa.org.uk*
International Surfing Association (ISA): *www.isasurf.org*
Academy of Surfing Instructors (ASI): *www.academyofsurfing.com*
Canal & River Trust: *www.canalrivertrust.org.uk*
Seaful: *www.seaful.org.uk*
Planet Patrol: *www.planetpatrol.co*
2 Minute Foundation: *www.beachclean.net*
Clare Osborn: *www.clareosborn.com*
Water Skills Academy: *www.waterskillsacademy.com*
SUPfm podcast: *www.supfmpodcast.com*
SUP Hub NI podcast: *www.suphubni.com*
SUP Mag UK: *www.standuppaddlemag.co.uk*
SUP International magazine: *www.sup-internationalmag.com*
Surfers Against Sewage: *www.sas.org.uk*
The Rivers Trust: *www.theriverstrust.org*
The Royal National Lifeboat Institution: *www.rnli.org*

Met Office: *www.metoffice.gov.uk*
BBC Weather: *www.bbc.co.uk/weather*
Tide Times: *www.tidetimes.org.uk*
Royal Life Saving Society UK: *www.rlss.org.uk*
Tide Times and Tide Charts: *www.tide-forecast.com*
Go Paddling: *www.gopaddling.info*
Ship Finder – The Live Marine Traffic Tracking App: *www.shipfinder.com*
SUPboarder magazine: *www.supboardermag.com*

Helpful apps
Windy: *www.windy.com*
Windguru: *www.windguru.cz*
Magicseaweed: *www.magicseaweed.com*
Paddle Logger: *www.paddlelogger.com*
RYA SafeTrx: *www.safetrxapp.com*
RiverApp: *www.riverapp.net*
WillyWeather: *www.willyweather.co.uk*
XC Weather: *www.xcweather.co.uk*
Ship Finder – The Live Marine Traffic Tracking App: *www.shipfinder.co*
Savvy navvy: *www.savvy-navvy.com*
Safer Seas & Rivers Service: *www.sas.org.uk/safer-seas-service*

Tracking your paddle
Paddle Logger: *www.paddlelogger.com*
RYA SafeTrx: *www.safetrxapp.com*
Strava: *www.strava.com*

Online safety courses
SUPfm podcast safety course: *www.supfm.thinkific.com*
Water Skills Academy iSUP Smart Course: *www.waterskillsacademy.com*

Acknowledgements

Writing this book has been a joy and privilege; an opportunity to explore some of the most beautiful places in Great Britain and meet wonderful paddle-boarders who so generously shared their time, knowledge and enthusiasm with me. I could not have done this without them:

Anu Aladin of Paddleboarding London, Katie Atherton of Cullercoats Collective, Steph Barnicoat and Percy, Simon Bassett of BSUPA, Tony Benton, Leanne Bird, Sarah Blackwell, Sarah Blues, Sid Whitney and Lucy, Imogen Broad, Patricia Carswell of Girl on The River, Alex Chester, Tara Crist, Caroline and Jonathan Dawson, Becky Dickinson, Chloe Drew, Anne Egan of SUP Mag UK, Michelle Ellison and Melanie Joe, Matt Gambles, Tristan Gooley, Karen Greenwood, Josh Haberfield, Emily Hague and Paul Hutchinson, Simon Hutchinson of SUPfm podcast, James Instance of Maritime and Coastguard Agency, Craig Jackson, Brian Johncey, Lisa Kenny, Cath Knight of Wye SUP, Michelle Lee, Ben Longhurst of Water Skills Academy, Donald Macpherson, Gemma Marshall, Adrian Mayhew of Surf Life Saving GB, Sue-Anne Mayne of SisterStay, Emily McLeod, Dr Adya Misra, Nicola Morgan of Puffin Dive Centre, Jojo O'Brien, Clare Osborn, Katie Owen and Fudge, Amira Patel of Wanderlust Women, Heather Peacock and her family, India Pearson, Dr Sarah Perkins, Brendon Prince, Nick Ray, Jayne Riggers, Oscar and the Liverpool SUP community, Sam Rutt, Clare Rutter, Gill Ryan, Catherine Sawyer, Sue Sayer and Charlie Gill of the Cornwall Seal Group Research Trust, Sean and Claire Scott, Ben Seal of British Canoeing, Alastair Smith, Mike Smith, Colin Speedie of WiSe, Jenny Spencer of British Canoeing, Mick Stockdale, Penny Stopher, Louise Sumner, Jo Taylor and Hayley Browning of the Paddlecabin, Tim, Kate, Jamie and the SUP Bristol community, Professor Mike Tipton, Linn van der Zanden, Cherie Whitby, Lucy Williams and Annabelle Yates.

Long before I spoke with Vertebrate Publishing, there have been people who, perhaps without realising it, gave me the confidence to believe my idea could become a reality. I am deeply grateful to them:

Bex Band of Love Her Wild, Matt Barr of Looking Sideways, Hannah Beecham and the RED January community, Poorna Bell, Di Binley, Tina Boden, Liv Bolton of The Outdoors Fix, Sam Bunch, Clare Carter, Emily Davis, Frankie Dewar, Martin Dorey, Dr Ruth Farrar of Shextreme Film Festival, Rhiane Fatinikun of Black Girls Hike, Alex Feechan and the FINDRA community, Deborah Garlick of Henpicked, Marina Gask of Audrey, Sarah Gerrish and Wonderful Wild Women, Jenni Godsland, Charlotte Graham, Nicky Green and the 2 Minute Foundation community, Jill Gregory Page, Cameron Hall of Holmlands, Kate Hardcastle, Alastair Humphreys, Anna Kessel of the Telegraph Women's Sport, Cadi Lambert,

Rachel Lankester of Magnificent Midlife, Alison Levett of the RNLI, Becky Lovatt and Emma Kitchen, Jackie Lynch, Hannah Maia of Maia Media, Cal Major and Lorna Evans of Seaful, Jo McEwan, Dr Juliet McGrattan and 261 Fearless, Harriet Minter and Antonia Taylor, Laurie Mucha of Feminista Film Festival, Helen Murray of Inside Tri Show, Mary-Ann Ochota, Rebecca Perkins, Rachel Peru of Out of the Bubble, Naomi Roberts of Canal & River Trust, Danielle Sellwood and Alex Rotas of Find It Film, Shelby Stanger of Vitamin Joy, Anne Stephens, Frit Tam of Passion Fruit Pictures, Lesley Tate of the Craven Herald, Alan Taylor of SUP North UK, the This Girl Can campaign, Colin Thunhurst and Leeds and Liverpool Canal Society, James Wight and the Adventure Uncovered team, John Wilson and Bo of Lake District Paddleboarding, Emily Woodhouse of Intrepid Magazine and the Yorkshire Rows.

Thank you to Kirsty Reade, Jess McElhattan and the team at Vertebrate Publishing for your patience, expertise and trusting me with the opportunity to write this book.

I'm grateful to Will Vaughan at Bluefin SUP for kindly gifting me Grace, my 12-foot paddleboard, in 2019. Thank you to all the Bluefin SUP team.

I would like to thank Sarah Thornely of SUPjunkie for being such a support and cheerleader to me and the paddleboarding community.

To Jason Elliott, thank you for always being there in my corner encouraging, and very often stretching, my dreams.

Thank you to Tim and Charlie for endless walks, dark chocolate and cups of tea and believing in me when I doubted myself.

Thank you to my sister Jane for being the best role model as a writer. I hope Mum would be proud.

Thank you to Henry and Johnny for teaching me to be brave with my life. You will always be my greatest and most special adventure.

Thank you to my dad for sharing his deep love and respect for the sea, and for patiently watching me in the bay when I paddleboard. This is for you, Dad, with all my love.

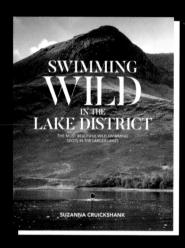
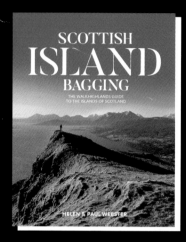
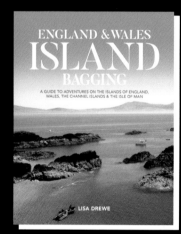
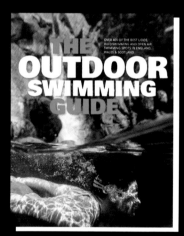

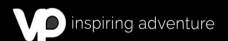